MENTAL DISORDER AMONG PRISONERS

MENTAL DISORDER AMONG PRISONERS

Toward an Epidemiologic Inventory

Nathaniel J. Pallone

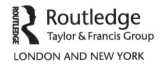

Routledge
Taylor & Francis Group

LONDON AND NEW YORK

First Published 1991 by Transaction Publishers

Published 2017 by Routledge
2 Park Square, Milton Park, Abingdon, Oxon OX14 4RN
711 Third Avenue, New York, NY 10017, USA

Routledge is an imprint of the Taylor & Francis Group, an informa business

Library of Congress Catalog Number: 90-11119

Library of Congress Cataloging-in-Publication Data

Pallone, Nathaniel J.
Mental Disorder Among Prisoners: Toward an Epidemiologic Inventory /
Nathaniel J. Pallone
    p. cm.
  Includes bibliographic references and index.
  ISBN: 0-88738-383-1
    1. Insane, Criminal and dangerous. 2. Mental illness — Epidemiology.
3. Violence — Etiology. 4. Prisoners — mental health services. I. Title.
RC451.4P68P34 1990
616.89'071—dc2090–11119
                                        CIP

ISBN 13: 978-0-88738-383-0 (hbk)

Contents

Preface

It is the burden of the volume to argue that — quite apart from any consideration of whether mental disorder is related "causatively" to the genesis of criminal behavior and quite apart from whether such disorder can be construed as exculpatory or not — such empirical evidence as is available suggests that the incidence of mental illness among members of correctional populations is substantially in excess of that found among members of the "general" population and that the high incidence of mental illness among such populations requires, merely for efficient management, the intervention of mental health professionals (e.g., for prisoner and staff safety in prisons) on a scale not yet seriously contemplated. Further, several decisions by the Federal courts and the U.S. Supreme Court suggest that prisoners have a right to mental health care; and we'd better get on with the task of providing that care, whether there is any reason to believe that by doing so we'll reduce recidivism or not. The clinical and operational issues are very real and, if we are to conform to what the courts have already constrained us to do, the implications for additional financial and professional resources are enormous.

But those are an epidemiologist's arguments that break little new conceptual ground. Instead, the conceptually engaging questions center around such issues as why we have set out to design a set of social policies that in essence dictate that one sort of deviancy shall virtually eclipse deviancies of other sorts — or, as the manuscript suggests, why we hold that deviancies are *not* created equal, whether in our constructions thereof *or* in the behavioral prescriptions that flow from those constructions.

In the interpretation of data from the neurosciences, I have benefited from the continuing assistance of Robert Pandina of the Center for Alcohol Studies at Rutgers, Kirtley Thornton of the Center for Health Psychology in South Plainfield, and Eugene Loveless of St. John's Hospital, Yonkers. James Hennessy of Fordham once again played the role of devil's advocate he has perfected in relation to my manuscripts these two decades. Joanne Williams continued her efficient ways in responding to my requests for research assistance. Adeline Tallau of the Library of Science and Medicine on the New Brunswick campus and Phyllis Schulze of the National Council on Crime and Delinquency at the Newhouse Center for Law and Justice on the Newark campus at Rutgers once again responded marvelously in helping me locate obscure references. Letitia, my spouse and partner, remained directly supportive and understanding of my peculiar work habits.

Nathaniel J. Pallone

1

Without Comprehensive Data, Bias Flowers Easily

On a given day in the United States, some 3,300,000 adults, or nearly 2% of the total population over the age of 18, are under the supervision of correctional authorities (Bureau of the Census, 1989, pp. 15, 184) as a result of conviction for criminal offenses. Of these, some two million are on probation, 550,000 are serving sentences in correctional facilities, and another quarter million are on parole (*Ibid.*, p. 184), while an additional 130,000 are incarcerated in jails while awaiting trial (Flanagan & Jamieson, 1988, p. 482). Collectively, they constitute the adult "correctional population."

Cherished Beliefs at Diametric Poles

In the absence of comprehensive data about the state of mental health in the correctional population, several cherished beliefs are afloat in the mental health and criminal justice communities concerning the extent of overlap between the "mad" and the "bad," to follow the disjunction popularized if not proposed by legal scholar Carol Bohmer (1976). An outrageous belief, deeply cherished among the "tender minded," holds that:

- All those who commit, or are convicted of, crimes (or at least of serious felony crimes, with "status" offenses like under-age alcohol consumption and similar behaviors that are at bottom merely *mala prohibita* but not really *mala in se* bracketed aside for the moment) are, virtually on the face of it, mentally ill. As a corollary, crime is itself the product of psychological disorder, frequently lubricated by biochemical disorder as well; from all of which it seems to follow that the appropriate "treatment" of offenders following conviction should emphasize rehabilitation and be guided by members of the mental health community.
- As a codicil, it is clear that, as we emptied the nation's mental hospitals over the past 25 years as a function of the advent of psychotropic

1

medication interacting with Federal social legislation in the form of the Community Mental Health Act of 1964, we filled its jails and prisons;[1] and the inescapable conclusion is that the prisons have become the repositories for a visible cadre of the mentally ill who are not "bad" and thus deserving of societal retribution through a punitive criminal justice system, but instead are "mad" and thus worthy of the ministrations of mental health care-givers.

- If you don't believe it, consider the case of Billie Boggs in New York, or go read maverick psychiatrist E. Fuller Torrey's (1988) scathing *Nowhere to Go: The Tragic Odyssey of the Homeless Mentally Ill*, which effectively portrays, to borrow Katharine Briar's (1983) phrase, correctional institutions as the new, and "neglected," asylums.[2] And consider the historic *Pugh v. Locke* decision in Mr. Justice Johnson's Federal District Court in Alabama (1976), which promised to reform the prisons of the nation by requiring not only humane housing and sanitary conditions but also "meaningful programs" staffed by qualified personnel and at least first-line mental health care within prison facilities, so that in the decade after *Pugh v. Locke,* dozens of states had been placed under Federal court order respecting one or another aspect of prison operation.

At the diametric extreme, there is an equally outrageous and equally cherished belief held by the "tough minded," to the effect that:

- The very concept of mental illness is an ever broadening and ultimately self-serving construction perpetrated on the public by psychiatrists and psychologists in order to make the necromancy they perform more palatable to fee-payers, including health insurance companies and the tax-paying public.
- As a corollary, the panoply of so-called "mental disorders" contained in the *Diagnostic and Statistical Manual of Mental Disorders* (Third Edition, Revised, no less), that massive lexicon of sorts and sources of unhappiness purveyed by the American Psychiatric Association, lists a wide array of conditions like "nicotine withdrawal" (coded at 292.00 in that volume) and "caffeine intoxication" (coded at 305.90) that no more deserve to be labeled "mental disorder" than the common cold deserves to be labeled a "physical disorder." And from that it follows that the appropriate "treatment" of offenders following conviction should emphasize retribution and deterrence; let the shrinks peddle their wares elsewhere.
- If you don't believe it, consider the wisdom of the Federal Congress in enacting the Kennedy-Thurmond Act of 1984, which effectively eliminated parole in the Federal prison system.[3] And don't forget that, in the 1988 elections, the "Get Tough, Hang 'Em High" presidential candidate who avowed wider application of the death penalty was overwhelmingly preferred over the candidate whose posture toward

prison furloughs bespoke at least an implicit belief in the prison as an institution the purpose of which is rehabilitation, or that regional and local candidates who embraced the same "Get Tough" posture by endorsing mandatory custodial sentencing for all sorts of felony crime were similarly preferred.[4]

The "Penrose Effect"

As in any cherished belief, a kernel of truth is to be found beneath each diametric polarity.

Half a century ago, British psychologist Lionel Penrose (1939) reported a neatly inverse relationship between the number of prison beds and the number of mental hospital beds across the nations of Europe in the 1930s; a quick reading of contemporary data might suggest that what has been called the "Penrose Effect" (Conacher, 1988) is alive and well in the United States (Brown & Smith, 1988; Kramer, 1977). According to data from the National Institutes of Health, the number of beds in public and private mental hospitals declined nationally from 451,000 in 1965 to 177,000 in 1985. According to Bureau of Justice Statistics data, during roughly the same period the number of convicted offenders confined in state and Federal prisons increased from 210,000 in 1965 to 420,000 in 1983, not including in either case those confined in jails or on probation or parole.

In an exhaustive review of the then-current research literature, Teplin (1983), although complaining about methodological flaws (perhaps inevitable, because research in this domain does not readily lend itself to the random assignment of "otherwise similar" subjects to such categories as offender vs. non-offender), concluded that "the research literature offers . . . support for the contention that the mentally ill are being processed through the criminal justice system." In part on the basis of his own earlier research (Lamb & Grant, 1982), distinguished psychiatrist H. Richard Lamb (1988, p. 1147) of the University of Southern California attributes the process whereby mental illness is criminalized to the confluence of a variety of psychological, social, and economic factors:

> As a result of deinstiutionalization, there are now large numbers of mentally ill persons in the community. At the same time, there is a limited amount of community psychiatric resources, including hospital beds. Society has a limited tolerance of mentally disordered behavior, and the result is pressure to institutionalize persons who

need 24-hour care wherever there is room, including jail. [The result is] a criminalization of mentally disordered behavior — a shunting of mentally ill persons in need of treatment into the criminal justice system.

That process leads to a cadre of "revolving door clientele" (Pallone & Hennessy, 1977) in jail facilities especially, whose crimes are relatively minor and who are generally released at trial, with their sentences reduced to "time served," after which they return to the same social circumstances from whence they came prior to their incarceration, so that, as Adler (1986) put it, "jails [become] a repository for former mental patients".[5] Such evidence may be relevant to the matter of the relative incidence of the "mad" among the "bad," but it fails to support the correlative contention that mental illness is criminogenic.

Contrary Data: New Facilities for Mental Health Care

To the contrary, it is also the case that we had created some 197,000 "places" in governmentally-supported alcoholism and substance abuse treatment units nationwide by 1985 that simply did not exist 20 years earlier. Absent data which detail what proportion of the 451,000 mental hospital beds (or the 177,000 prison beds, for that matter) of 1965 were occupied by patients or inmates with alcohol or substance abuse disorders, it is of course impossible to correlate these data definitively; but it is a reasonable speculation that the apparent decline in treatment provision for the mentally ill has not been quite so dramatic as an initial reading of the data might suggest. Moreover, during the same period, we had created a network of governmentally-sponsored community mental health centers designed to provide at least first-line mental health care *in situ* and short of psychiatric hospitalization that simply did not exist in 1965.

Recent empirical studies provide scant support for either side of the controversy over the obverse question — i.e., the relative incidence of the "bad" among the "mad." Thus, in an investigation of homeless adults, Gelberg, Linne & Leake (1988) reported that subjects who had previously been psychiatrically hospitalized indeed were frequently involved in subsequent criminal activity and tended toward a high frequency in drug and alcohol abuse. In sharp contrast, Phillips, Wolf & Coons (1988), in a study of 2735 previously hospitalized schizophrenics in Alaska over a four-year period, found that only 0.2% to 2.0% were arrested each year for violent crimes, with these arrests accounting for only between 1.1% and 2.3% of annual arrests for all violent crimes in that state.

Toward Sophisticated Guesswork

It is easy to dismiss these polarized biases as clearly simplistic, the product of feverish brains that have particular axes to grind. A more moderate approach might grant that some portion of those who commit serious crimes are indeed *seriously* mentally disordered, quite apart from whether a specific mental disorder is related to the particular criminal behavior at hand in any way that can reasonably be said to be "causative."

That more moderate approach might also grant that mental disorders, like physical disorders, come in a variety of shapes and sizes and degrees of severity, some of which, like *both* the common cold *and* caffeine intoxication, are essentially self- curable (if not indeed self-limiting) *and* that people who are seriously mentally ill should be accorded the opportunity for appropriate treatment for their illness, whether that illness is "causative" of criminal behavior, antecedent to criminal behavior, or even engendered subsequently (perhaps as a function of the sanctions imposed for that behavior), in much the same way that dental treatment for an abscess is accorded to even the most cold-blooded predator meritorious of the most severe punishment, even when one is absolutely certain that to withhold such treatment can itself be construed as punitive.

Yet there is no readily accessible body of data that are responsive to the issue of the relative incidence of serious mental illness among those who have been convicted of criminal behavior, whether such illness can be construed as causative or not. Were it the case that a comprehensive census had been taken of the mental health status of the more than three million citizens in correctional custody, on parole, or on probation on a given day in any recent calendar year, one would court little truck with cherished beliefs.

But, despite more than two decades of fairly careful and reasonably scientifically sophisticated data-gathering about an incredible array of sometimes minute aspects of the criminal justice and correctional systems and despite the fact that at least a cursory and untutored categorization of an offender's mental health history is now routinely included in the recommendation made by a probation department in many jurisdictions relative to sanction before sentence is imposed, no such enumerative census yet obtains.

Nonetheless, fragmentary data are available in a wide variety of studies. These data can be consolidated to form a picture that is strongly suggestive, if not quite definitive. The process of consolidation requires a degree of guesswork, with the resultant estimates more or less sophisticated, varying in accordance with the scientific validity of the data bases from which one extrapolates, but also, if truth be told, with the cherished beliefs of whoever is doing the extrapolating and the degree of tough mindedness or tender mindedness brought to the task.

The Burden of Inconvenient Knowledge

In a marvelous passage in his epic *Western Star,* Stephen Vincent Benet portrays a meeting between John Brown, that "rude frontiersman drunk on God," and a group of northern liberals led by William Lloyd Garrison of the *Boston Liberator* who are to finance assault by Brown and his sons on the Federal garrison at Harper's Ferry. Brown is anxious to describe in detail the technical ingenuity reflected in his plan to scale the palisades of the Potomac. But Garrison and his cohorts decline to hear the tale: "Pray, sir, do not burden us with inconvenient knowledge."

The most egregiously tender minded, consistent with their conviction that all criminal behavior is the product of mental disorder, will doubtless see the failure to develop a comprehensive mental illness census of the correctional population as the result of a deep desire to avoid the burden of inconvenient knowledge. As sociologist Walter Gove (1982) has proposed, if we avoid labeling those among the "bad" who deserve to be called "mad," we simultaneously avoid the prescriptions for our own behavior that flow from that second label.

Yet it may be eminently arguable that the adequate "management" of correctional populations, whether in correctional facilities or through probation and parole systems, would seem to require a relatively accurate estimate of the extent of mental illness — and particularly of those varieties of mental illness related to explosive or disruptive behavior—among those in custody or whose behavior is presumably to be monitored, even when such illness cannot be construed as exculpatory or even as particularly related to criminal behavior in any manner than can be called "causative." In that sense, lack of comprehensive data about the characteristics of members of correctional populations would seem to ill serve even the "Get Tough" crowd. Thus, Steadman, Rosenstein, MacAskill & Mandersheid (1988) have recently complained that, "[i]n developing public policy and designing appropriate services for persons who intersect the mental health and criminal justice systems, one of the major impediments has been the absence of even basic descriptive data."

One might suspect that the failure to commission enumerative mental health census surveys of the correctional population, in a society which is still quite schizoid in its thinking about what behavior to regard as deviant, about what behavior to label psychiatrically deviant and what behavior to label criminally deviant, and especially about the extent to which mental illness should serve to exculpate or merely to explain criminal behavior, might in some fashion be predicated on an understandable desire to avoid the burden of "inconvenient knowledge." However that may be, the fact is that two exhaustive studies of the characteristics of incarcerated offenders undertaken by the U.S. Bureau of the Census for the Department of Justice — covering jail inmates in the first instance (1980) and prison inmates in the second (1988) — paid scant attention to the mental health status of respondents while focusing very heavily on patterns of drug and alcohol use.

Further, beyond a first impression that mental health census-taking should represent a relatively easy undertaking among members of a population whose freedom is judicially restricted (an impression that for several technical reasons may prove rather too glib, however, since a comprehensive mental health evaluation that meets contemporary standards for thoroughness may require detailed neurological inquiry as well), there lurk a number of rather significant sets of impediments concerning the issue of whether current mental status at the time of the criminal behavior itself or at the time of the census-taking should be the focal concern.[6] If the former, one either is required to accept retrospective self-reports or to attempt to amass corroborating evidence from external sources. If the latter, one is left with the question of whether current status at the time of the census-taking itself is in any reasonable way indicative of a prior pattern or emerged as an artifact of confinement. From the perspective of the tasks of managing correctional populations, however, it is the latter and only the latter that holds operational significance.

Notes

1. It is instructive to recall that Mr. Justice Johnson, who handed down the decision in *Pugh v. Locke* in 1976, the historic case that created the precedent under which the prisons of many states were to be reformed by order of the Federal courts in the following decade, also handed down the *Wyatt v. Hardin* and *Wyatt v. Stickney* decisions of 1971, upheld by the Supreme Court four years later in the landmark case that reformed the mental hospitals of Alabama and, by extension, of the nation, by affirming the right of patients to treatment and establishing standards to govern the ratio between patients and professional staff as well as a panoply of

other aspects of hospital operation. And it is even more instructive to note that, between 1970 and 1976, as benchmarks for assessing the impact of the *Wyatt* decisions, the budget for the mental hospitals of Alabama had increased by 230% while the patient population had decreased by 58%, with the "unserved" segment apparently diverted from inpatient to outpatient treatment via a network of community mental health centers not subject (or perhaps not *yet* subject) to judicially-imposed standards for patient care (Pallone, 1986, pp. 33–35; Stickney, 1976; Windle, Poppen, Thompson & Marvelle, 1988).

Nor is the phenomenon localized. In a review of the compliance of the various states with the Federal Mental Health Systems Act of 1980 which followed the *Wyatt* decisions, with a particular focus on implementation of the rights of patients, Brown & Smith (1988) found that only when the inpatient populations in mental hospitals *declined* did the states implement the rights of the *reduced* cadre of inpatients served. The investigators comment (pp. 162, 164): "There is little evidence to suggest that [implementation of] these rights was the direct outcome of humanitarian or liberal beliefs about the way mental patients ought to be treated."

2. Long before Torrey penned his indictment of the wrong- headedness inherent in a national social policy of de- institutionalizing the mentally ill that, in effect, "liberated" the seriously dysfunctional from the back wards of public mental hospitals but consigned them instead to outpatient treatment in under-funded community mental health centers staffed largely by grossly overloaded, underpaid sub-professional mental health clinicians (abetted, to be sure, by liberal prescriptions for, if not dosages of, psychoactive medication), National Public Radio produced in 1980 *Catch Me If You Can* (with perhaps a hint or two from O. Henry), a dramatic rendition that encapsulates the conventional wisdom marvelously.

The central figure is a girl diagnosed as schizophrenic in childhood, with the hint that the disorder is attributable to unspecified anomalies in brain biochemistry. She graduates from placement in special education classes in childhood to private residential treatment facilities in adolescence. After the death of her parents, she enters the process of revolving-door admissions to and discharges from public mental hospitals, where she is confined on average for six weeks, "stabilized" on medication, then remanded to "aftercare" in a community mental health center.

Once discharged, she only intermittently avails herself of such outpatient treatment and routinely, in what has become the classic revolving-door pattern, fails to take the prescribed medication, which has the effect of "robbing" her, however temporarily, of the symptoms to which she has become accustomed and with which she feels comfortable. At her last admission to a state hospital, a compassionate psychiatrist despairs of the network of social policies that virtually require her discharge from a structured environment in which, because she is under a mantle of protection (if not paternalism) and well-ordered control, she is able to function at a level that is "more nearly normal" than the bag-lady life she lives outside the institution. The psychiatrist induces her to set fire to the blanket on her hospital bed, thus destroying public property maliciously. Now, of course, she is eligible to become a client of the criminal justice system, which is able to provide for her, via incarceration in a women's prison, a similarly protective, structured, well-ordered environment — but for a three-year period rather than for the six weeks accorded her as a client of the mental health system.

3. Curiously, half a decade after enactment of Kennedy-Thurmond, the Federal courts operate under constraint of a set of criminal sentencing guidelines which, by design, recapitulate the parole decision guidelines operative in the Federal prisons for the dozen years prior to enactment of that legislation (von Hirsch, 1988; Block & Rhodes, 1990).

4. During the same elections, the same electorate again largely declined to support the issuing of public debt bonds to finance the construction of prison facilities to house those offenders who are the focus of just such policies, let alone disdaining the increased taxes required to support the staffing of those facilities on an annual basis. Thus, though the number of offenses and the number of jurisdictions subject to mandatory custodial sentences increases apace, the population of the nation's prison facilities grows but modestly each year; nor, in the face of Federal court constraints interacting with the refusal of the taxpayer to approve construction of new facilities, could one reasonably expect otherwise.

As if to compensate, new and technologically advanced methods of electronic surveillance of probationers (and, in some jurisdictions, of parolees) have been introduced, holding promise to relieve (whether by explicit design or by fortunate effect matters little) what would otherwise prove to be intolerable overcrowding in the prisons and jails likely to result in yet other Federal court orders. Yet, as Morris & Tonry (1990, p. 3) have eloquently argued, even these new "intermediate community sanctions" lack credibility: "Judges, prosecutors, and the general public too often simply don't believe intermediate punishments are effective."

Nonetheless, whether by design, by happenstance, or as a sort of subliminal compensation for enacting "Get Tough" laws, other legislation (e.g., that governing the processing of alcohol and drug users in many states through pretrial intervention programs) permits some offenders who are both formally guilty of criminal behavior and psychiatrically (or biochemically) disordered to be diverted from the criminal justice system into the mental health "system," even when the essential features of their disorder(s) can provide no basis for exculpation by the stringent criteria for the insanity or the "diminished responsibility" defenses — with the effect that prison populations remain relatively stable while the roster of those offenders, whether convicted or "diverted" prior to conviction, for whom responsibility has been shifted to the mental health community rises dramatically.

5. As Briar (1983) has commented: "The anti-institution movement in recent decades has prompted the de- institutionalization of dependent populations (e.g., delinquent youths, the mentally ill, the developmentally disabled, alcoholics); the jail has emerged as a repository for such persons. The great diversity of jail populations exacerbates the inability of jail staff to handle inmates effectively, resulting in service deficiencies that increase the likelihood that the inmate becomes damaged as a result of jail time."

Scull (1984) has put the case even more pungently: "The shift away from a social control apparatus placing heaviest emphasis on segregating deviants into institutions like asylums [has] displayed remarkably little resemblance to liberal rhetoric on the subject. Indeed, the primary value of that rhetoric . . . seems to have been its usefulness as ideological camouflage, allowing economy to masquerade as benevolence and neglect as tolerance . . . for many ex- inmates and potential inmates, the alternative to the institution has been to be herded into newly emerging deviant ghettos, sewers of human misery and what is conventionally defined as social pathology, within which society's refuse may be repressively tolerated."

6. Indeed, even the validity of instruments customarily used to assess scientifically mental health or illness has been called into question when these instruments are applied to members of offender populations. Thus, McGovern & Nevid (1986) studied the impact of experimentally-manipulated "cues" about the use to which results of the Minnesota Multiphasic Personality Inventory would be put on the responses of some 120 incarcerated sex offenders. Those subjects who had been "positively cued" (i.e., led to believe that positive self-disclosure would be considered indicative of psychological health) demonstrated significantly higher scores on the F scale (generally held to be indicative of candor and/or defensiveness as test-taking attitudes) and significantly lower scores on the K scale, generally held to be indicative of a deliberate attempt to portray oneself unfavorably (Greene, 1988; Walters, White & Greene, 1988). Simultaneously, these subjects also reported significantly greater symptoms of anxiety on the Hopkins Symptom Checklist.

2

Epidemiological Studies of Mental Health and Illness

Few would expect the level of mental health among members of the correctional population to *exceed* that among members of the general population. In the absence of comprehensive data, however, there is simply no valid way either to confirm or disconfirm a proposition that seems on its face unlikely. Nor, however, is there a valid way either to confirm or disconfirm that the rates of mental illness found in epidemiological studies of the general population are not univocally applicable to members of the correctional population as well.

Methods of Assessing Mental Disorder

The nearly 240 distinct mental disorders detailed in the American Psychiatric Association's (1987) current lexicon can be divided into what are usually called the *functional psychological disorders* (defined as those without identifiable etiology in central nervous system, brain, or physiological functioning) and the *neuropsychiatric disorders* (that is, those whose etiology can be traced to anomalies or impairments in neurophysiological functioning or which result in impaired physiological functioning). The functional disorders include conditions as diverse as compulsive personality, recurrent depression in the absence of external stimuli objectively sufficient to elicit depressive reactions, and free-floating anxiety, similarly in the absence of sufficient external stimuli. The neuropsychiatric disorders include conditions as diverse as psychogenic pain, anorexia, impaired sexual performance, and dementia arising from the inexorable process of aging or from damage to the brain caused by accident, stroke, or habituation to alcohol or drugs. A further and very useful distinction made by the psychodynamicists categorizes disorders as "ego-syntonic" (those which are accepted by the person who suffers them as part and parcel of his or her usual ways of behaving — compulsivity, for example — and therefore do not

11

engender a subjective sense of discomfort) *or* as "ego-dystonic" (those which are perceived as alien to the self and therefore trigger subjective discomfort).

Differential Diagnosis for Disorder-Specific Treatment

Especially since the explosion in the availability of psychoactive medication, much of it designed to relieve or at least obviate the more virulent effects of specific disorders (technically, groups of disorders) which are usually accompanied by subjective distress, contemporary scientifically-anchored practice in the mental health professions requires *differential* diagnosis as the essential first step in the treatment of mental disorder — that is, to apply disorder-specific treatment, whether psychotherapeutic or pharmacotherapeutic, it is necessary not merely to determine that the prospective patient is "abnormal" in some way but to identify the specific character of such abnormality. In the optimal situation, the differential diagnostic process will also specify the etiology of the disorder or disorders to be treated (i.e., whether they arise from faulty patterns of nurturance and interpersonal learning, from disordered neuropsychological functioning, or from some combination of contributing factors).

The diagnostic process typically involves an assessment of the prospective patient's current mental status (i.e., present level of functioning), a review of his or her social and developmental history (often taken from the self-reports of the patient, but verified through independent sources whenever possible), and the administration of one or more carefully constructed, and thus presumably scientifically sound, psychometric diagnostic instruments. Clearly, since it involves the investment of substantial professional person- power, the diagnostic process is time-consuming and labor- intensive.

From another perspective, the diagnostic process preparatory to disorder-specific mental health treatment can be construed as the application of a series of screens with ever finer mesh to information about the prospective patient. The first screen, with a rather gross mesh, merely establishes whether he or she experiences subjective discomfort or whether, in relation to others to whom he or she can reasonably be compared, he or she exhibits disorders in thinking, feeling, or behaving; the final screen, with the finest mesh, determines the *specific way or ways* in which the prospective patient is disordered, resulting in a differential diagnosis and, optimally, an indication of etiology as well. In actual practice, the first and least fine screen has usually been applied during the process of referral, by self or by others, before the prospective patient initially encounters the examining clinician.

Epidemiological Survey Techniques

Expressed somewhat simplistically, the goal in medical epidemiology is to determine both the means by which physical disease (or illness) is transmitted and those groups who are particularly at risk. In the first case, medical epidemiology relies on the investigative methods of the biological sciences and, in the second, on those of the social sciences. These basic investigations are generally preparatory to the energizing of public health efforts to control the spread of illness or disease, through what is sometimes called "preventive medicine." At the level of the control of illness or disease, the development of a statistical portrait of members of those groups empirically determined to be at particular risk (or, in the more familiar terminology associated with infectious medical disorders, "susceptible") is paramount. "Risk factors" may be found to inhere in genetic or constitutional predisposition, environmental influences (e.g., exposure to toxins), and/or "lifestyle" variables. A current example which has engaged both medical epidemiologists and public health officials, no less than energized the public, is the control of Acquired Immune Deficiency Syndrome (AIDS), *both* by stemming its spread in the population (largely through efforts to convince members of "at risk" groups to alter their behavior) *and* by developing pharmacologic agents that will alter the course of the disease once the disease has been contracted.

Analogously, the goal in *psychiatric epidemiology* has been to identify those groups statistically at greatest risk for mental and emotional disorders of various sorts (Mechanic, 1980, pp. 54–72) in relation to a variety of external stressors and/or predictive factors. A current example is the effort to identify those persons who are at risk inter-familially and/or inter-generationally for alcoholism and, again, the preventive measures pivot largely on efforts to convince "at risk" groups to alter their behavior.

Epidemiological studies of mental health and illness, which owe their origins more to public health than to mental health professionals, generally tolerate screening procedures with less than a fine mesh. From the public health perspective, in order to plan treatment facilities and services appropriately it may arguably be more important to determine the proportion of the population that, in the aggregate, suffers from mental disorder of *any* sort than it is to know the relative frequency with which disorders of specific sorts can be discerned — that is, to

13

know *that* a person is mentally disordered in some unspecified way than to know through differential diagnosis in what specific way or ways he or she is disordered.

A countervailing argument can be made, however, that disorder-specific treatment, and especially disorder-specific pharmacotherapeutic treatment, absolutely requires knowledge of the relative frequency with which disorders of specific types afflict member of target populations and that, in the absence of such information, even so elemental a public health function as manpower planning to identify the type and number of treating professionals — e.g., M.D. psychiatrists vs. Ph.D. psychologists vs. master's-level social workers or rehabilitation counselors — required to address such disorders cannot proceed on a rational basis. Nonetheless, epidemiological studies of mental disorder have come to rely on investigative methods that fall short of approximating the professional diagnostic process.

The earliest epidemiological investigations typically did no more than enumerate the diagnoses assigned by treating professionals to successive admittees to psychiatric hospitals or to other mental health service facilities (Lemkau, 1961; Burke & Regier, 1988), with the obvious limitations in respect of non-patients. Other studies (e.g., Pasamanick, 1962) selected random, stratified samples representative of the community in which the study was conducted, then undertook careful, professional diagnostic evaluations of subjects. While this method, which in effect replicates the differential diagnostic process, doubtless produces data more readily interpretable to the mental health community, it is so labor-intensive as to engender prohibitive costs.

More typically, epidemiological studies have been conducted in the community at large (often on a door-to-door basis) by means of interview schedules consisting largely of questions about symptoms of mental illness, designed to be administered by non-specialists in mental health and relying principally or exclusively on the self-reports of respondents. Although the resulting data lack the specificity of formal diagnoses assigned by mental health professionals, even when subjects' questionnaire responses are later reviewed by professional clinicians (in a sort of long-distance, hands-off, third-party analogue to a formal diagnostic procedure) before the subject is categorized as mentally healthy or ill, it is this method that has become standard in psychiatric epidemiological studies (Orvaschel, Sholomskas & Weissman, 1980; Shrout, Lyons, Dohrenwend et al., 1988; Weissman, Myers & Ross, 1986).

The Fineness of the Mesh in the Screen

Adoption of this methodology among epidemiologists has not been without controversy, however. As distinguished medical sociologist David Mechanic (1980, pp. 45–46) has observed, this method of inquiry produces what may be construed as rather a gross "screen," through which many disorders might be expected to pass undetected:

> [I]nterview measures . . . for screening persons in community populations . . . tend to include items measuring depression, anxiety, and psychophysiological discomforts but not psychotic symptoms or antisocial behavior. They focus more on *neurotic* distress than loss of reality . . . The value of such global measures of psychiatric impairment and their appropriate use have engendered much critical debate.

Or, as the psychodynamicists might put it, the research methodology typical in epidemiological studies seems sensitive primarily to those functional disorders that are ego-dystonic—and hence readily identifiable by respondents in consequence of subjective distress. And it seems unlikely, except in gross circumstances (e.g., memory loss caused by recent and very readily identifiable brain injury), that the neuropsychiatric disorders, and especially those that are ego-syntonic (e.g., impulsivity predicated on brain-bioelectrical anomalies) can be identified by self-report in the absence of discerning professional assessment.

Nonetheless, the eminent social psychiatrist Leo Srole has defended the methodology (Srole & Fischer, 1986, pp. 83–84) by contending, in essence, that a gross screen is all that is required for mental health census purposes:

> The symptom questions [are] chosen to represent the manifest currents of behavioral disturbance that generally reflect the emotional substrate underlying most of the many narrowly circumscribed patient syndromes to which psychiatrists try to attach a specific diagnostic tag . . . the sample of symptoms covered [is] intended not for the impossible task of discriminating among those numerous syndromes (especially in cases falling outside the clinical range of full blown pathology, as most do), but to mark, as does a physician's thermometer, progressive grades of deviation in emotional "fever" and disability, from an asymptomatic state of presumptive wellness.

If applied to physical illness, that argument might be interpreted to suggest that it is epidemiologically unnecessary to know whether elevated body temperature is triggered by a minor and self-limiting ailment like the common cold or signals a pervasive systemic infection, even though the former likely requires only rest and perhaps over-the-counter medication selected and administered by the patient, while the latter clearly requires the intervention of professional medical personnel. Since mental illnesses also come in a variety of shapes and sizes, some essentially self-limiting and others requiring professional intervention, Weissman, Myers & Harding (1978, p. 459) have complained that the "gross screen" approach simply is not discerning enough to produce useful data and further reveals a rather too simplistic conceptualization of a common etiology for disorders of varying shapes and sizes:

> Psychiatric epidemiology in the United States has been dominated for the past 30 years by the view that mental illness is unitary and [that] various diagnostic [categories] represent different manifestations of the same underlying defect in mental functioning . . . Community surveys have assessed frequency of overall impairment . . . rather than rates of specific psychiatric disorders. Consequently, there are no recent data on rates of . . . specific psychiatric disorders based on community surveys in the United States.

To remedy that situation, Weissman and her colleagues at Yale devised a more discerning approach to the construction of mental health census screening instruments with a finer mesh, more closely approximating a clinical interview in mental health practice, and, not incidentally and somewhat surprisingly, yielding ratios of mental illness in the general population generally negatively discrepant from those revealed by the earlier gross screen methodology.

Studies of Mental Illness in the General Population

Whatever the specific methodology, more than half a century of research in psychiatric epidemiology has consistently indicated that clear symptoms of serious mental illness — defined approximately to coincide with the disabling psychoses, including those of organic origin, the more severe neuroses, significant mental retardation, and certain personality pattern disturbances that incline the individual toward an "explosive temperament," usually resultant in aggressive behavior, with the aggregate set requiring professional mental health attention—are found in the general population in a relative frequency ranging from 11% to 37%. The ratios reflect, but do not appear to be governed by, the fineness of the mesh in the screening devices. Simultaneously, these studies have rather consistently identified a portion of the general population as entirely symptom-free and a mid-range group that exhibits symptoms of "mild" mental illness.

Gross Screen Studies

In their well-known *Mental Health in the Metropolis* study, Srole, Langner, Michael, Opler & Bennie (1962) utilized a gross screen procedure. Data were gathered through in-home interviews conducted by non-specialists, following a schedule of questions designed to elicit subjects' self-reports about "120 manifestations of mental disturbance." Srole and his associates found that 22% of their sample were so mentally or emotionally disordered as to require professional intervention, with 59% mildly disordered and only 19% symptom-free. In a second survey undertaken 20 years after the original study, Srole & Fischer (1986) found 33% to be seriously disordered, 25% to be symptom-free, and 42% to be mildly disordered.

Similarly, levels of mental disorder judged severe enough to warrant professional attention were found in 20% to 30% of respondents studied in rural towns in eastern Canada by Leighton, Leighton & Armstrong (1968), again with only 19% symptom-free; among 29% of those studied by Wheaton (1982) in New Haven, with 28% symptom-free and with 42% with mild or moderate symptomatology; and among 32% of subjects in New York studied by Williams, Endicott & Spitzer (1986), with 28% entirely symptom- free.

In Chicago, Ilfeld (1978) found a "high" prevalence of what he terms *psychiatric* symptoms among 15% of his subjects, "moderate" symptomatology among another 25%, and "low" symptomatology among the remaining 60%, with none of his subjects symptom-free. Ilfeld also reported that 24% of his subjects reported one or more *psychosomatic* disorders, with the two categories not mutually exclusive. A substantially higher proportion, at 37%, of mental disorder was found among subjects followed longitudinally in Iceland by Helgason (1986).

Fine Screen Studies

In a "fine screen" investigation conducted in 1936 but recapitulated in a more recent retrospective analysis, Lemkau (1986) found that 24% of the subjects in his Baltimore sample exhibited symptoms of mental disorder sufficient to warrant professional attention, 19% exhibited symptoms of mild disorder, and 43% were symptom-free. Conducted at the Johns Hopkins School of Hygiene and Public Health, this investigation relied on analyses by mental health professionals of the medical records of subjects in addition to assessments of their questionnaire responses.

In another study set in Baltimore that involved "thorough clinical and laboratory evaluations at the Johns Hopkins Hospital" rather than relying on self-reports from subjects and that was conducted as a joint research venture of the American Medical Association, the American Public Health Association, and the American Public Welfare Association, Pasamanick (1962) found a rate of mental disorder serious enough to warrant treatment of only 11%.

In the Yale epidemiological series developed around a "fine screen" approach to non-clinician interviews, Weissman, Myers & Harding (1978) found evidence of mental disorder at a level of severity warranting intervention in 18% of their New Haven subjects, with 82% symptom-free; both ratios were replicated in another study in the Yale series by Myers & Weissman (1986).

In what has perhaps been the most ambitious and surely the most carefully designed mental health census yet undertaken, psychiatric researchers Burke & Regier (1988) at the National Institute of Mental Health have reported data from the NIMH Epidemiologic Catchment Area Program for five cities, involving a total sample of nearly 19,000 respondents selected to accurately represent the national population. Subjects were interviewed using the Diagnostic Interview Schedule (DIS) developed at NIMH (following the general methodology advocated by Weissman and her associates) to reflect specific diagnostic criteria for the major groups of mental disorders contained in the American Psychiatric Association's *Diagnostic and Statistical Manual*; the DIS has been incorporated into the diagnostic process in routine clinical practice, so that a "running census" of patients, at least in Federally funded mental health installations, is now possible. As a further validity check and to ascertain what proportion of subjects had sought treatment subsequent to the first interview, respondents in the NIMH studies were re-interviewed six and twelve months later. The prevalence of mental disorder was found to be 19%, including 9% who evinced anxiety disorders, 6% with substance use disorders, and 1% each with schizophrenic disorders, cognitive impairment, or anti-social personality disorder (*Ibid.*, p. 82). Data from the relevant studies, arrayed by the fineness of the screening procedure, are recapitulated in *Figure* 1.

Figure 1. Proportions of the General Population Judged to be Seriously Disordered, Mildly Disordered, or Symptom-Free in Mental Health Epidemiological Studies.

Screen Mesh/Source	Serious Disorder	Mild Disorder	Symptom Free
Gross Screen			
Srole et al., 1962	22%	59%	19%
Leighton et al., 1968	30%	51%	19%
Ilfeld, 1978	15%	25%	0%
Wheaton, 1982	29%	42%	28%
Helgason, 1986	37%		
Srole & Fischer, 1986	33%	42%	25%
Williams et al., 1986	32%	40%	28%
Median	30%		
Fine Screen			
Pasamanick, 1962	11%		
Weissman et al., 1978	18%		82%
Lemkau, 1986	24%	19%	43%
Myers & Weissman, 1986	18%		82%
Burke & Regier, 1988	19%		
Median	18%		

Even though the NIMH Diagnostic Interview Schedule has now been widely adopted both in epidemiological studies and in clinical practice, questions remain about whether data gathered by non-clinician interviewers yield systematic underestimates of the overall prevalence of mental disorder. Psychologist Lee Robins (1985) of the Washington University School of Medicine, a principal architect of the DIS system, contrasted data to emerge from interviews conducted by well prepared non-clinicians using the Diagnostic Interview Schedule in Baltimore and St. Louis respectively with data based on clinical interviews with the same subjects conducted by psychiatrists at Washington University and at Johns Hopkins. Robins found a relatively consistent pattern, in which the prevalence of mental disorders as judged by psychiatrists generally exceeded that as judged from the results of interviews conducted by non- clinicians using even this well-constructed instrument that had been subjected to extensive validity analysis. Psychiatrists in St. Louis found evidence of panic disorders twice as often as lay interviewers, mania and depression three times as often, and phobia half again as often, but of schizophrenia only half as often; there were no differences in respect of alcohol, drug, or obsessive disorders. Psychiatrists in Baltimore found evidence of phobia, alcohol, and depressive disorders twice as often and of drug and obsessive-compulsive disorders three times as often, while non-clinicians found panic disorders eight times as often, with essentially no differences in schizophrenia or mania. Roughly congruent findings were reported by Erdman, Klein, Greist & Bass (1987), who contrasted the formal diagnoses assigned professionally to 220 psychiatric patients with categorizations resultant from non-clinician administration of the DIS.

However, the distinguished British medical sociologist George W. Brown (1986, p. 177) observed that what he called "more lenient" diagnostic practices in the United States may tend to inflate rates of mental disorder. And, in his inimitably incisive prose, Schofield (1986, p. 13) proposed that "The total incidence of mental illness in the population is greater during those periods in the national economy which support the expense of mental health census-taking than during economic periods that do not support such surveys" and, as a corollary, that "The greater the number of psychiatrists, psychologists, and other trained mental health experts in the population, the higher the incidence of mental illness."

Applying Median Rates to Correctional Populations

The median rate of serious mental disorder reported in epidemiological studies utilizing the gross screen methodology is 30%, and, in studies utilizing a fine screen, 19%. Since there is no particular reason to believe that the level of mental health among members of the correctional population is greater than among members of the general population, the tender minded observer might reasonably speculate that the incidence of mental disorder among the correctional population approximates 30%. If one adopts the more discerning "fine screen" approach of Lemkau, Pasamanick, Weissman and her colleagues, and the NIMH researchers, one would conclude that the incidence of mental illness among the general population is closer to 19% and thus the tough minded would *more conservatively* speculate that such a ratio will also obtain among members of the correctional population.

Either speculation would pivot, however, on two assumptions: that the correctional population mirrors the general population in important demographic characteristics and that mental disorder is not associated in any significant way with the criminal behavior on account of which a particular individual finds himself or herself a member of a correctional population.

Demographic Characteristics of Correctional Populations

Consideration of the comparative demographics which differentiate the correctional from the general population reveals that such an assumption encapsulates some serious flaws.

According to Bureau of the Census (1989, p. 15) data, 84% of the general U.S. population is white. According to data from the Federal Bureau of Justice Statistics as reported in the mammoth *Sourcebook of Criminal Justice Statistics* (Flanagan & Jamieson, 1988, p. 491), only 49% of state prison inmates and 66% of Federal prison inmates are white, with racial composition among jail inmates, probationers, and parolees not reported. Similarly, Census data indicate that nearly 51% of the general population is female, while the *Sourcebook* reports that only 4% of state prison inmates and 6% of Federal prison inmates are female. In relation to their proportion in the general population, non-whites are over-represented on a ratio greater than 3:1 in the Federal prisons and on a ratio greater than 4:1 in the state prisons; women are under-represented at a ratio of 12:1.

Even though precise comparative data is not available, it seems a reasonable speculation that the prison population is skewed in the direction of the lower socioeconomic classes; nor, in view of the complexities between race and socioeconomic class in the United States, should one expect otherwise. Thus, Bureau of the Census data (1989, p. 38) indicate that only 12.5% of U.S. workers earn less than $9999 per year, but the *Sourcebook* reports that fully 60% of the inmates of state prisons had an income below that level in the year preceding incarceration (Flanagan & Jamieson, 1988, p. 494). Similarly, Census data report that only 24% of the general population had completed fewer than 12 years of formal education, while *Sourcebook* data indicate that 53% of state prison inmates had completed fewer than 12 years of education.

Demographically, then, state and Federal prison inmates, two major segments of the correctional population, are disproportionately male and non-white in comparison to the general population; state prison inmates are drawn primarily from that segment of the larger society at the lowest levels of education and income. These factors suggest caution in extrapolating to the correctional population mental health and illness ratios derived from stratified samples (which can be expected to reflect sex and race ratios and socioeconomic status in correct proportions) of the general population.

What is known about differential rates of mental illness among non-whites, among males, and among members of lower SES groups? Will such knowledge yield a more sophisticated guess about the relative incidence of mental disorder among the correctional population than univocal predication of the prevalence ratios derived from epidemiological studies of the general population?

Relative Incidence of Mental Disorder by Race

Two studies at Johns Hopkins, each utilizing a fine screen methodology, are the earliest investigations of differential rates of mental disorder among whites and non-whites.

Lemkau's (1986) inquiry, conducted in 1936 but recapitulated in a recent retrospective analysis, found that the non-white subjects in his metropolitan Baltimore sample exhibited symptoms of psychoneurosis 158% as often as white subjects and of psychopathic personality disorder 127% as often. In the second study, Pasamanick (1962) found that non-whites experienced organic brain disorders an astounding 720% as often as whites and significant mental deficiency 161% as often as whites. However, non-whites were found to experience psychoses only 75% as often as whites and psychoneuroses only 44% as often. In view of the massive discrepancy in the incidence of organic brain disorders and the large discrepancy in the incidence of mental deficiency, the overall differential ratio reported by Pasamanick — i.e., that whites experience serious mental disorder 174% as often as non-whites — masks some important contrasts in focal symptomatology that are of particular significance to those interested in criminal behavior and/ or charged with the management of correctional populations. Ilfeld (1978), however, found essentially no differences in the prevalence either of what he terms psychiatric or psychosomatic disorders by race among his Chicago subjects. More recently, Myers & Weissman (1986), in a longitudinal study over a ten-year period in New Haven, found that non-whites experienced depressive symptomatology only 61 % as often as whites and pathological grief reactions only 49% as often; no comparisons by race were reported with respect to other diagnostic categories, nor to organic brain disorders or mental deficiency. Radloff & Locke (1986) similarly reported that current, as distinct from lifetime, symptoms of depression were experienced by non-whites only 88% as often as by whites in a sample of Kansas City residents, again with no data concerning other diagnostic categories, organic brain disorders, or mental deficiency.

Utilizing a variant methodology, Warheit, Bell, Schwab & Buhl (1986) studied the incidence not of particular diagnoses but rather of what they called "psychosocial dysfunction" among 4200 residents of southeastern states, reporting that such dysfunction at a level requiring professional attention was found among non-whites 138% as frequently as among whites. Derived from a factor analysis computed by the investigators, the "psychosocial dysfunction" measure is said to assess "the behavioral consequences of psychiatric symptomatology rather than symptoms alone".[1] *Figure 2* recapitulates data from these studies.

In the aggregate, with the exception of Lemkau's pioneering study of 50 years ago and Ilfeld's Chicago study, these investigations seem to suggest a differential ratio between non-whites and whites such that *non-whites experience what are generally called "functional psychological disorders"* (i.e., those without identifiable etiology in central nervous

Figure 2. Relative Frequency with Which Selected Symptoms of Mental Disorder Were Observed among Non-white and White Subjects in Mental Health Epidemiological Studies of the General Population.

Symptom	Source	Non-White/ White Ratio
"Functional" disorders		
Depression	Myers & Weissman, 1986	*0.61*
	Radloff & Locke, 1986	*0.88*
Grief, pathological	Myers & Weissman, 1986	*0.49*
Psychiatric disorder	Ilfeld, 1978	*1.07*
Psychoneurosis	Pasamanick, 1962	*0.44*
	Lemkau, 1986	*1.58*
Psychopathic personality	Lemkau, 1986	*1.27*
Psychosis	Pasamanick, 1962	*0.75*
Psychosocial dysfunction	Warheit et al., 1986	*1.38*
Neuropsychiatric disorders		
Mental deficiency	Pasamanick, 1962	*1.61*
Organic brain syndrome	Pasamanick, 1962	*7.20*
Psychosomatic disorder	Ilfeld, 1978	*0.90*

system, brain, or physiological functioning) *less frequently than whites; but* it also appears to be the case that *non-whites experience what are generally called "neuropsychiatric disorders" (organic brain disorders, mental deficiency) more frequently than whites*[2] and that significant psychosocial dysfunction is encountered more frequently among non-whites than among whites.

Relative Incidence of Mental Disorder by Gender

Relevant data concerning the differential incidence of mental disorder among males tend to be scattered and fragmentary and are often embedded virtually as "incidental" information in studies that focus on other variables. Thus, Lemkau's (1986) study of fifty years ago found that adult males experienced symptoms of psychoneurosis only 64% as often as adult females; Murphy (1986), in a retrospective analysis of data from the studies undertaken in the 1950s by the Leightons and their associates in eastern Canada, found "major psychiatric disorder" to be only 57% as prevalent among males under 45 as among females in the same age group and to be only 44% as prevalent among males over 45 as among similarly-aged females.

Ilfeld (1978) reported that men suffer symptoms of psychiatric disorder only 42% and of psychosomatic disorder only 45% as often

Figure 3. Relative Frequency with Which Selected Symptoms of Mental Disorder Were Observed among Male and Female Subjects in Mental Health Epidemiological Studies of the General Population.

Symptom	Source	Male/Female Ratio
"Functional" disorders		
Depression	Myers & Weissman, 1986	*0.52*
	Radloff & Locke, 1986	*0.79*
Grief, pathological	Myers & Weissman, 1986	*0.17*
Major psychiatric disorder	Ilfeld, 1978	*0.42*
	Murphy, 1986 (Ss aged 45−)	*0.57*
	Murphy, 1986 (Ss aged 45+)	*0.44*
Psychoneurosis	Lemkau, 1986	*0.64*
Psychosomatic disorder	Ilfeld, 1978	*0.45*
Psychosocial dysfunction	Warheit et al., 1986	*0.58*

as women; Myers & Weissman (1986) found lifetime depressive symptomatology only 52% as often and symptoms of grief reactions only 17% as often among males as among females; Radloff & Locke (1986) found current symptoms of depression among men only 79% as frequently as among women; and Warheit, Bell, Schwab & Buhl (1986) found significant psychosocial dysfunction only 58% as frequently among men as among women. The relevant data are recapitulated in *Figure* 3.

In the aggregate, these investigations seem to suggest that a differential ratio obtains between males and females such that *men experience "functional psychological disorders" less frequently than women;* but the data are essentially silent with respect to differential ratios in "neuropsychiatric" disorders.

The Issue of Socioeconomic Class

Data concerning the relative prevalence of mental disorder inflected by socioeconomic status (SES) prove even more elusive than similar data inflected by sex. Thus, Lemkau's (1986) early Baltimore study and Myers & Weissman's New Haven study (1986) found only tiny differences among and between varying SES groups in the focal disorders they investigated. But both Ilfeld (1978) and Radloff & Locke (1986) found the highest levels of current depressive symptomatology among the lowest income groups and the lowest levels among the highest income groups, both among blacks and among whites, while Warheit, Bell, Schwab & Buhl (1986) found a neatly inverse geometric progression between SES and relative frequency of significant psychosocial dysfunction, such that such dysfunction was encountered nearly twice as often in the lowest as in the highest SES group.

In their classic study *Social Class and Mental Illness,* Hollingshead & Redlich (1958) focused on the twin issues of the differential diagnoses assigned by clinicians for similar symptomatology when experienced by members of varying SES groups and on the character of professional treatment accorded to members of those groups for such disorders, reporting that the neuroses were the modal diagnoses for members of the middle and upper classes, that the psychoses were the modal diagnoses for members of the lowest classes, and that the rate of mental illness per 100,000 of the population was greatest in the lowest SES group, by a factor nearly treble the rate in the highest SES groups (pp. 171–219). Those general trends were confirmed in a recent study by Gift, Strauss, Ritzler & Kokes (1988) at the University of Rochester

Hospital, who added that the "greatest interclass difference occurred between the lowest and the adjacent social class." Similarly, Toch, Adams & Greene (1987) found evidence of the "Hollingshead Effect" among prison inmates categorized by ethnic background.

Further, both in their original monograph and in a recent retrospective analysis of their work of 30 years earlier, Hollingshead (1986) reported, virtually as incidental data, that *the criminal justice system itself (i.e., police and the courts) represented the modal source of referral to treatment for members of the lowest SES group* (i.e., the group with the highest rate of disorder) with symptoms either of neurosis or psychosis. In the aggregate, these data may be relevant primarily because they suggest that mental disorder among members of the lower socioeconomic groups is likely to remain undetected and untreated until an act of putatively criminal behavior triggers referral to a professional source of assistance.[3]

Psychometric Studies among Prisoners

It has already been observed that a formal diagnosis is the essential first step to contemporary clinical practice in the mental health professions and that the diagnostic process typically involves a clinical assessment of the prospective patient's current mental status, a review of his or her developmental history, and administration of one or more validated psychometric diagnostic instruments. The first two elements provide an ipsative cross-sectional picture of the patient and his or her current functioning, while the third element provides a comparative view of the patient in relation to others of his or her age, race, and/or sex.

The MMPI as a Clinical and Research Tool

The psychometric instrument most frequently employed to fulfill the latter function is the Minnesota Multiphasic Personality Inventory (MMPI), the psychometric device that has been characterized in no less a source than the American Psychiatric Association's "official" *Textbook of Psychiatry* as the instrument- of-choice for the differential diagnosis of current mental disorder (Clarkin & Hurt, 1988, pp. 229–231).

Structurally, the MMPI consists of some 566 statements, with a fourth-grade reading level, which subjects endorse as True or False of themselves. So far, the instrument looks not very different from the interview schedules used in epidemiological studies, although the genealogy is quite the reverse — i.e., the MMPI preexisted all but the earliest such interview schedules, and indeed those developed for the studies of Srole and his associates (1962, 1986) selected some of their items from those of the MMPI. But the resemblance ends there, for, through a sophisticated psychometric process called "criterion referencing," the *pattern* of responses given by each subject is compared to those of members of the standardization sample whose psychiatric diagnoses were established through exhaustive formal diagnostic procedures conducted by mental health professionals, so that the resulting "scores" reflect the degree of congruence between a given subject's self-reports and those of members of distinct diagnostic groups whose differential diagnoses have been firmly established by customary intensive professional examination (Anastasi, 1988, pp. 526–530; Graham, 1987, pp. 4–5). The instrument thus provides a very "fine screen" indeed for the identification of psychopathological conditions.

The Ten Primary Clinical Scales

The instrument yields scores on three measures of what has been called "test-taking attitude," including dissimulation, and on ten "primary clinical" scales: *Hypochondriasis*, or abnormal preoccupation with physical complaints; *Depression; Hysteria*, or the tendency to translate emotional problems into physical symptoms; *Psychopathic deviation*, or the tendency toward disregard of customary social mores; *Masculinity-femininity*, or the tendency to endorse traditionally opposite-gender-linked interests and attitudes; *Paranoia; Psychasthenia*, or obsessive rumination coupled with compulsive behavior; *Schizophrenia; Mania*, or elevated mood and accelerated speech and motor activity; and *Social introversion*, or the tendency to withdraw from social contacts and responsibilities. Over the course of the years, some 132 additional or "derivative" scales have been developed (Graham, 1987, pp. 116–194), in the main also on a criterion-referenced basis (e.g., the MacAndrew Alcoholism Scale).

A score equivalent to the 97th percentile (represented by a value of 70 on the normalized "T" distribution on which scores are reported) constitutes the customary threshold level for assessment of serious disorder in professional mental health diagnosis; this point is usually called the "threshold of clinical significance." In the early days of the instrument's use, index codes representing the two or three highest scales (and often the lowest one or two as well) were employed to describe configural patterns for subjects (Hathaway & Meehl, 1956), but this practice has more recently yielded to computerized scoring and profile interpretation. Essentially a self-administering, paper- and-pencil device, the MMPI is incapable of directly detecting neuropsychiatric disorder, brain syndromes, or mental deficiency except at the most profound (non-reader) level. Nonetheless, the MMPI is sensitive to a number of characteristics (e.g., psychopathic deviation, mania, schizophrenia, psychasthenia, social introversion) which *may*, in given cases, represent behavioral manifestations secondary to underlying neuropsychiatric disorder amenable to psychometric inventory, as several investigations to be reviewed in Chapter 4 suggest.

In addition to its ubiquity in clinical practice, the MMPI is very likely the most widely researched diagnostic instrument in history; by Anastasi's (1988, p. 526) count, it had been the subject of some 8000 investigations in the half-century following its publication, with additional studies accumulating at the rate of 250 per year (Maloney & Ward, 1979, p. 312). A decade ago, a major restandardization study to provide contemporary norms inflected by age and sex was undertaken at the Mayo Clinic (Colligan, Osborne, Swenson & Offord, 1989).

The MMPI in Studies of Criminal Offenders

Because of its wide use clinically and the ever expanding research data base, it is not surprising that the MMPI has been employed extensively in studies of criminal offenders (Gearing, 1979). Most often, these studies have focused on determining the patterns that differentiate offenders who have been convicted of crimes of one sort from those convicted of crimes of other sorts or from comparison subjects never convicted of any offense (e.g., in studies by Blackburn, 1975, and Jones, Beidelman & Fowler 1981, of violent and non-violent offenders; Holcomb & Adams 1982, of white and non-white murderers; Lindgren, Harper, Richman & Stebbens, 1986, in differentiating recurrent and non-recurrent delinquency; McCreary, 1976, in investigations of assaultive and non-assaultive male and female offenders; Panton, 1977, 1978, 1979, on drug dealers vs. abusers and on offenders who sexually assault adults or children violently and non-violently respectively; and Walters, Scrapansky & Marlow, 1986, on offenders in the military).

Though no enumerative mental health census of the correctional population has been undertaken with the MMPI, fragmentary and instructive data are found in a number of studies; a few have focussed directly on the question of the relative incidence of mental health and illness in offender samples (e.g., Walters, 1986), but most have reported relevant data incidental to other focal concerns.[4]

The Megargee-Bohn Typology Study

In the ambitious undertaking which yielded a new and exemplary psychometric model for the classification of offenders useful both in program planning and in decisions about security classification levels, Edwin Megargee of Florida State University (who had earlier made important contributions to the understanding of criminally assaultive behavior that eventuated in the development of an MMPI scale to measure "over-controlled hostility," as described by Megargee in 1966, Megargee, Cook & Mendelsohn in 1967, and Megargee & Cook in 1975) and Martin Bohn of the Federal prison system analyzed in detail MMPI data on 6350 inmates of Federal prisons, including 1350 who were followed throughout the period of their incarceration and subsequent to release.

Extensive analysis yielded a typology of ten distinct offender groups with characteristic MMPI profiles, with which specific patterns of criminal behavior and distinct social history variables were found to be statistically associated (Megargee, 1977; Megargee & Bohn, 1977; Megargee, 1986). The Megargee-Bohn typology has been cross-validated in a number of studies, including those by Edinger (1979) on a large sample of prisoners (1291 males, 146 females) in state correctional facilities; by Edinger, Reuterfors & Logue (1982) on adult males in a forensic mental health unit; by Henderson (1983) on non-violent offenders; by Smith, Silber & Karp (1985) on women inmates; by Veneziano & Veneziano (1986) on juvenile offenders; by Walters (1986) on offenders in the armed forces; by Dahlstrom, Panton, Bain & Dahlstrom (1986) on death row inmates; by Mrad, Kabacoff & Duckro (1983) on paroled offenders in halfway houses; and by Megargee (1986) on prisoners who had threatened to assassinate the president.

In a review of the accumulated research evidence, Zager (1988) concluded that "the reliability, validity, and practical utility of the system have been demonstrated." That is not to say, however, that no jarring sounds have been heard.

One of the principal purposes that guided the Megargee-Bohn typology study was the development of a system for the classification of inmates according to the level of security supervision required; along with MMPI data, data from a panoply of other sources were analyzed, and the typology of ten offender groups (with colorful designations, like "Easy" and "Foxtrot") was empirically derived. Some investigations have questioned the universal applicability of the Megargee-Bohn typology to offender populations in such specialized settings as halfway houses (Motiuk, Bonta & Andrews, 1986) and medium security facilities like prison camps (Baum, Hosford & Scott, 1984), or for *post*dicting lifetime criminal violence (Moss, Johnson & Hosford, 1984). Megargee himself has questioned the predictive validity of several derivative scales concerning prison adjustment constructed from the initial typological data (Megargee & Carbonell, 1985); Louscher, Hosford & Scott (1983) and Kennedy (1986) have similarly questioned the effectiveness of the typology in predicting inmate aggression; and Johnson, Simmons & Gordon (1983) have questioned the stability of the typology over time. In contrast, however, Villanueva, Roman & Tuley (1988) reported that the typology accurately *post*dicted rehabilitation outcome among offenders in a residential treatment facility. These findings, however, vitiate neither the validity of the source data nor the process of reassembling of those data into a mental health census format.

Re-assembling the Megargee-Bohn Data in Census Format

Because their principal monograph is rich in its presentation of source material (Megargee, Bohn, Meyer & Sink, 1979, pp. 107–138), it is possible to reassemble the Megargee-Bohn source data so as to represent an approximation to a mental health census of their sample, and to do so in a manner that mimics one important aspect of the professional diagnostic process. Because the data emanate from a scientifically sound, criterion-referenced diagnostic instrument, the process clearly represents the application of a very "fine screen." *Figure* 4 recapitulates the re-assembled data by reporting the proportions of the Megargee-Bohn subjects who score above the clinical threshold level on each scale,[5] while *Figure* 5 recapitulates these data by reporting the proportion of those subjects who score above that threshold on various combinations of MMPI scales.

It has already been observed that, in clinical practice, psychological disorder is typically assessed through score elevation on one or more of the ten "primary clinical" scales at a T-value of 70, equivalent to the 97th percentile. By this criterion, fully 74% of Megargee & Bohn's subjects are classifiable as psychologically disordered — a ratio dramatically in excess of any found in epidemiological studies of the general population, at more than double the median figure for studies utilizing a "gross screen" approach and greater by nearly four-fold than the median for studies utilizing a "fine screen" approach. Only 26% of the Megargee-Bohn subjects exhibited no score on the ten clinical scales above the

Figure 4. Proportion of the Megargee-Bohn Federal Prisoner Sample Scoring Above the Critical T-Value of 70 (97th Percentile) on Each of the MMPI Primary Clinical Scales.

MMPI Scale	Proportion Above T = 70
Hyphochondriasis	*13%*
Depression	*20%*
Hysteria	*13%*
Psychopathic deviation	*58%*
Masculinity-feminity	*0%*
Paranoia	*22%*
Psychasthenia	*25%*
Schizophrenia	*24%*
Mania	*37%*
Social introversion	*0%*

threshold level, thus constituting an analogue to the "symptom-free" group in general epidemiological studies. Further, these "symptom-free" subjects also demonstrated "criminal behavior patterns at the milder end of the continua" and tended to have abused illicit drugs with lower frequency as well.

That high proportion is *not* inconsistent but instead accords closely with the level of mental disorder among prisoners reported in a substantial number of studies which have employed a wide variety of assessment modalities with a less discerning screen mesh than the MMPI.

Thus, Gormally, Brodsky, Clements & Fowler (1972, pp. 21, 67–69) reviewed unpublished studies reviewed on psychiatric evaluations of 1700 felons admitted consecutively to the central state prison in North Carolina, which found only 5% without identifiable mental disorder and 20% with "transient" disorder, and on 32,500 military prisoners, which found only 21% to be free of mental disorder. Similarly, distinguished psychiatrist Marc Schuckit and his colleagues at the School of Medicine of the University of California, San Diego (Schuckit, Herrman & Schuckit, 1977) found evidence of what they called "formal psychiatric illness" through "structured personal interview" rather than through psychometric assessment among 46% of newly arrested offenders *without* prior convictions, while another 27% evinced drug or alcohol use disorders, so that mental disorder conditions classifiable under the rubrics of the American Psychiatric Association's *Diagnostic*

Figure 5. Proportion of the Megargee-Bohn Federal Prisoner Sample Scoring Above the Critical T-Value of 70 (97th Percentile) on Combinations of the MMPI Primary Clinical Scales.

Combination/Grouping	Proportion Above T = 70
On one scale or more	74%
On one scale or more, excluding *Pd*	60%
On two scales or more	57%
On two scales or more, excluding *Pd*	33%
On three scales or more	33%
On three scales or more, excluding *Pd*	33%
On four scales or more	22%
On five scales or more	13%
On Paranoia, Schizophrenia, *or* Mania	50%
On Paranoia, Schizophrenia, *and* Mania	13%
On (Paranoia, Schizophrenia, *or* Mania) *and Pd*	30%
On Paranoia *and Pd*	22%
On Schizophrenia *and Pd*	21%
On Mania *and Pd*	34%

and Statistical Manual were discerned in a total of 73% of their sample *without* application of a "fine screen" device like the MMPI.[6] Walters, White & Greene (1988) likewise reported that only 22% of their sample of Federal inmates were found to be free of mental disorder on the basis of non-psychometric clinical assessment of case history and interview information.[7] In studies among juvenile offenders, McManus, Alessi, Grapentine & Brickman (1984) reported that 100% of their sample of delinquents had received "multiple psychiatric diagnoses" on the basis of psychiatric interviews conducted through the use of a forerunner of the NIMH Diagnostic Interview Schedule.

High Scale Combinations in the Megargee–Bohn Data

Consideration of the proportions of offenders in the Megargee-Bohn sample who score above the clinical threshold level on a single scale may be too liberally literal a reading, yielding unrealistically high proportions of mental disorder. In clinical practice, a score beyond the threshold of clinical significance is not held to be equally indicative of severe disorder on each of the ten primary scales; an elevated score on the masculinity-femininity scale, for example, does not carry the same clinical weight as a score of similar elevation on schizophrenia, mania, or paranoia. Instead, active psychopathology sufficient to warrant professional intervention (whether through inpatient or outpatient treatment) is typically assessed through an even "finer screen" that usually considers abnormally high — and mutually confirmatory — elevations on two or more scales.

Further, because the psychopathic deviation scale was initially criterion-referenced on a sample that included adjudicated offenders (McKinley & Hathaway, 1956, pp. 98–103), one is tempted to bracket aside scores on the scale which measures psychopathic deviation (*Pd*) as redundant with the defining characteristic of an offender population; even so, it is surprising that 42% of the Megargee-Bohn subjects do *not* exceed the clinical threshold level on this scale.[8]

With the exclusion of those who are "merely" psychopathic, the proportion of subjects who reach the clinical threshold on one or more scales reduces to 60%. If one focuses only on those subjects whose scores reach this threshold on one or more of the three scales held to be indicative of the most severe psychopathology — viz., the scales that measure paranoia, schizophrenia, and mania, respectively — and still excludes the *Pd* scale, the proportion of offenders who surpass the clinical threshold level reduces to 50%, still substantially in excess of ratios reported in general epidemiological studies. Indeed, if one attends only to scores on the scale which measures mania, it is the case that 37% of the Megargee-Bohn sample meets or exceeds the threshold level, a ratio that exceeds for a single disorder (albeit a troubling disorder from the perspective of correctional management and/or law enforcement as well as that of a theory of criminogenesis) the ratios found in general epidemiological studies for all disorders combined, except among Helgason's subjects in Iceland.

But, particularly within a correctional context, it may be argued that an individual who is *both*, say, paranoid *and* psychopathic presents quite a different set of management problems than one who is "merely" paranoid — and so on, through the various combinations of an elevated reading on psychopathic deviation *plus* an elevated reading on one of the three scales that measure the severest and, putatively, most disabling forms of psychopathology.

In the case of paranoia combined with psychopathic deviation and of schizophrenia combined with psychopathic deviation, the ratios in the reassembled Megargee-Bohn data exceed the median "fine screen" ratio for all disorders combined reported in the Yale and NIMH studies and meet the ratio for all disorders combined reported in Srole et al.'s original "gross screen" study; in the case of mania combined with psychopathic deviation (a conjunction that, as Holland, Beckett & Levi [1981] have reported, is frequently found among offenders convicted of crimes of violence) the ratio for the reassembled data exceed the "fine screen" ratios by nearly two-fold.

Especially since the Diagnostic Interview Schedule developed for the Epidemiological Catchment Area studies has now entered "mainstream" clinical practice and will very likely become a standard record-keeping approach in mental health installations, a final comparison can be made between the reassembled Megargee-Bohn psychometric data and comparable figures from the consolidated NIMH interview data (Burke & Regier, 1988, p. 83). Relevant data are recapitulated in *Figure* 6. The discrepancies are so astoundingly large, ranging from prisoner/general population ratios of 300% in the case of depression to 2600% in the case of schizophrenia, between the incidence of mental disorder as inferred from data gathered by non-clinicians in the first instance and as psychometrically inventoried in the second, as to speak for themselves.[9]

Interpretation with Caution

In interpreting these data from the Megargee-Bohn study, it should be noted that the populations of Federal prisons differ substantially from those of state prisons with respect to the character of offense. Thus, according to *Sourcebook* reports, only 29% of Federal prisoners are serving sentences for crimes of violence (McGarrell & Flanagan,

Figure 6. Relative Frequency with Which Selected Mental Disorders Were Observed among Respondents in the NIMH Epidemiological Catchment Studies (Burke & Regier, 1988) and among Prisoners in the Reassembled Megargee-Bohn Data.

Disorder	Prisoners	NIMH Subjects
Depression	*20%*	*6.3%*
Mania	*37%*	*0.5%*
Obsessive-compulsive disorder	*25%*	*1.5%*
Psychopathic deviation	*58%*	*0.8%*
Schizophrenia/Schizophreniform disorder	*24%*	*0.9%*
Somatization disorder/Hysteria	*13%*	*0.1%*

1985, p. 665), while 57% of state prisoners are serving sentences for violent crimes (p. 657). If serious psychological disorder is, as may be inferred from the Megargee-Bohn data, less rarely encountered among offenders whose criminal behavior falls near the "milder" polarity, and if it is the case that offenders confined to state prisons differ from Federal prisoners precisely in that their criminal behavior falls near the "harsher" polarity, it may well be that the Megargee-Bohn proportions represent systematic *under*estimates of the prevalence of psychological disorder among the latter (and larger) segment of the correctional population.

Mental Retardation among Prisoners

Significant mental retardation of such character as to render the person unable to appreciate the nature of his or her behavior is a prime empirical determinant for exculpation for the responsibility for criminal behavior under the M'Naghten Standard (West & Walk, 1977) for insanity prevalent in the criminal codes of the various states. In a well-ordered world, in which criminal defendants availed themselves of the defenses open to them, one would expect to find virtually no mental retardates among the prison population; instead, one would expect such offenders to be confined in forensic psychiatric institutions.

Nonetheless, in a survey among prison administrators in 48 states, Denkowski & Denkowski (1985) found that mentally retarded inmates constituted 2% of the prison population. The operational definition for assessment of mental retardation was set as an IQ below 70 on the Wechsler Adult Intelligence Scale, Revised, the standard threshold on the psychometric measure of intelligence standard in clinical practice. In consequence of the psychometric specificities of the Wechsler instrument in relation to the normal probability distribution, one would anticipate finding some 2.27% of the general population below an IQ level of 70 (Anastasi, 1988, pp. 90, 252), so that the prevalence rate for prisoners reported by Denkowski & Denkowski is slightly (and, very likely, not significantly) *lower* than chance expectancy for the general population. Nonetheless, McAfee & Gural (1988, pp. 7–8) believe that the proportion of mental retardates among imprisoned offenders reported by Denkowski & Denkowski is artificially low, since "Identification of defendants with mental retardation is more than haphazard in most states" and "defendants with mental retardation who are quiet, cooperative, and 'normal' in appearance may never be assessed" formally.

Figure 7. Relative Frequency with Which Mental Retardation Was Observed among Respondents in Epidemiological Studies of the General Population and among Prisoners in the Denkowski & Denkowski (1986) Data.

Disorder/Source	Prisoners	Non-Prisoners
Cognitive impairment, Burke & Regier, 1988		1.3%
Mental deficiency, Pasamanick, 1962		1.5%
Mental retardation, Denkowski, 1986	2.0%	

Persons who are severely mentally retarded (some 0.13% of the general population, with IQs below 55 on the Wechsler) continue to be confined in institutions for the care of retardates (Landesman & Butterfield, 1987). Perhaps for this reason, few epidemiological studies of mental health and illness in the general population have assayed the prevalence of mental retardation. Pasamanick (1962) fixed the ratio at 1.5% on the basis of detailed examination of his subjects at Johns Hopkins Hospital and further observed that the incidence was greater among non-whites than among whites at a ratio of 161% [*Figure* 2]. In the NIMH Epidemiological Catchment Area studies based on the Diagnostic Interview Schedule, Burke & Regier (1988) report the rate of "severe cognitive impairment" at 1.3%.

According to the Denkowski & Denkowski data, *the prevalence of psychometrically-inventoried mental retardation in the prison population exceeds that found in the general population*, whether by Pasamanick's psychometric methods (at a ratio of 133%) or through non-clinician interviews (in the NIMH studies, at a ratio of 154%). The relevant data are recapitulated in *Figure* 7. While these ratios are not astronomical, they are the more surprising since mental retardation itself constitutes the grounds for exculpation under the M'Naghten Standard.[10]

The Limits of Generalizability

Information about the probable relative incidence of mental disorder among prisoners very likely cannot be generalized to the "universe" of criminal offenders. Given markedly low rates of apprehension and conviction, there is every reason to believe that those incarcerated in correctional facilities are *not* representative of those who commit criminal offenses. Further, there are good reasons to believe that offenders who are placed on probation differ from those sentenced to prison in ways that are directly relevant to the status of their mental health.

Imprisonment as an Infrequent Consequence to Crime

Comprehensive data of national scope on the proportion of crimes committed that result in conviction and sentence to the intrusive sanction of imprisonment are not available (Flanagan & Jamieson, 1988, p. 411). To assemble data that respond to these concerns requires tracking individual cases through a number of pathways and into succeeding years: Criminal activity may be reported in one year, a suspected offender arrested and an indictment placed (or the charge dismissed) in a second year, and trial held (in consequence of various delays in preparation of the case, location of witnesses, and the like) in a third year.

In the absence of comprehensive data, however, the *Sourcebook of Criminal Justice Statistics* (Flanagan & Jamieson, 1988, pp. 411–413) reports the results of a "pilot study" of the consequences of felony arrest in eleven states selected to resemble the nation in important demographic characteristics; collectively, the eleven states account for 38% of the national population and 37% of the episodes of *reported* crime. When the data on sequelae to arrest are read in juxtaposition to data on the incidence of felony crime reported in these jurisdictions for the relevant years *(Ibid.,* p. 319), the picture that emerges strongly resembles the "funnel effect" observed in the President's Commission Report (1967, p. 61) of more than two decades ago.

Thus, for every 1000 crimes reported in these jurisdictions, there were only 207 arrests. Each 207 arrests led to 49 decisions to release the arrestee without prosecution. Of the each remaining 158 arrestees, 4 were acquitted at and 154 convicted. Of each 154 convicted, 59 were sentenced to prison and 95 were sentenced to probation. These data are graphically recapitulated in *Figure* 8.

If it is the case that each of the 1000 reported crimes has been committed by a single offender without replication (an unlikely situation), then a data set (fragmentary or otherwise) which represents at maximum only 59 of 1000 offenders (i.e., those who are incarcerated and thus accessible as subjects in psychological investigations) could hardly presume to speak for the total offender population. Unless it be the case that the overwhelming majority of those offenses which are reported but which are not correlated with subsequent arrests are committed by those who are arrested and charged (also an unlikely condition, given usual police practices in aggregating charges), it is arguable that the overwhelming majority of offenses are committed by offenders who are never apprehended, let alone prosecuted and convicted.

Figure 8. Imprisonment as an Infrequent Consequence to Crime — For Every 1000 Crimes Committed, There Are Only 154 Convictions, With 95 Sentences to Probation and 59 Sentences to Prison (Flanagan & Jamieson, 1988).

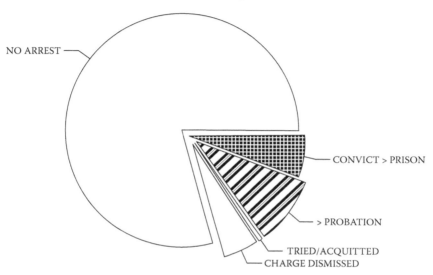

One may reasonably speculate that evasion of apprehension is not a random behavior; rather, it is more likely the product of careful planning. That requires a modicum of what Warheit, Bell, Schwab & Buhl (1986) have designated psychosocial competence, which they regard as the obverse of the consequences of mental disorder. Thus, it may well be the case that the incidence of mental disorder among those offenders who are never apprehended is substantially lower than among than those who are. To the extent that psychosocial competence of this sort requires a higher degree of mental health (not to say also, of functional intelligence, as Kunce, Ryan & Eckelman [1976] observed), it may be the case that the very act of apprehension serves as a mental health screen.

It may also be a matter of more than passing interest that a substantial discrepancy obtains in racial distribution between arrestees and prisoners, such that 71% of all arrestees but only 49% of state prison inmates are white (Flanagan & Jamieson, 1988, pp. 378, 494).

The Probation Report as a Screening Device

In cases in which there is judicial discretion in sentencing (in some jurisdictions for some offenses, prisons terms are mandatory), the offender's prior record is assuredly a determinant of incarceration. Hence, it is likely that the majority of those offenders sentenced to prison terms are not "first offenders," while the obverse obtains for those sentenced to probation.

In the typical circumstance, the decision on sentence is made by the presiding judge after receiving the report of a probation officer responsible to the court concerning the character of the accused, his or her prior involvement with the criminal justice system, economic status, family obligations, standing in the community, the likelihood of satisfactory completion of probation as an alternative to incarceration, and other factors likely to influence the court's decision in the matter of incarceration vs. probation (Frishtik, 1988).

Among the criteria to which probation officers explicitly attend are those which correspond to the principal empirical referents of "psychosocial dysfunction" as defined by Warheit, Bell, Schwab & Buhl (1986). To the extent that those criteria reflect the consequences of mental disorder of a severe character, the process of probation review itself serves to screen *out of* the prison population those convicted offenders whose work, economic, and family situations have not been overtly disrupted as a consequence of mental disorder or otherwise; and, to the same extent, that review serves to screen *into* the prison population those offenders in whom the incidence of "psychosocial dysfunction" is virtually by definition disproportionately high.[11]

Indeed, in a massive study at the RAND Corporation of nearly 15,000 sentencing decisions in California a decade earlier, Klein, Petersilia & Turner (1990, p. 815) reported that a history of drug or alcohol use (itself constituting a mental disorder, as discussed in Chapter 3) made a potent contribution to judicial choice of probation rather than prison as a sanctioning option; thus, in this case, evidence of mental disorder served to screen offenders *into* prison. Other potent contributors identified were those principally reflective of competence in avoiding the consequences of criminal behavior: prior prison terms or juvenile incarcerations, commission of the instant offense while on probation or parole for a prior offense. The use of a weapon during the instant offense was also related to the sanctioning decision to imprison — as also were the fact that the defendant was *not* represented by a private attorney (but instead appeared *pro se* or was represented by a public defender) *and* that the defendant chose to avail himself or herself of the right to trial by jury rather than entering a plea of guilty.[12]

However, the race of the defendant was found to make only a tiny contribution to the sentencing decision,[13] accounting for only one percent of the variance, so that the investigators were able to conclude that "California courts are making racially equitable sentencing decisions" (p. 816) and, implicitly, that "[there are] more blacks in prison [not] because of racial bias in the criminal justice system [but] because they are more likely than whites to commit those crimes that lead to imprisonment" (p. 812). The finding that race is not a factor contributing to the sentencing decision contrasts rather sharply with results reported by Pruitt & Wilson (1983), in a study of sentences over a ten year period in Wisconsin, and by Peterson & Hagan (1984), in a study of sentences over a 13-year period in New York. Moreover, the RAND study does not inquire into why it might be the case that non-whites "are more likely than whites to commit those crimes that lead to imprisonment." Pasamanick's finding that, although non-whites suffer functional psychological disorders less frequently than whites, the prevalence of organic mental disorder is more prevalent at a ratio of 720% may be relevant, particularly when read in juxtaposition to data that link such disorder to neurogenic criminal violence, to be reviewed in Chapter 4.

Conclusion

Demographic differences between the prison population and the general population indicate that the former are disproportionately male and non-white. It is to be anticipated, therefore, that the prevalence and specific character of mental disorder found among imprisoned offenders will be congruent with the differential incidence and specific character among males and among non- whites in the general population. Data extrapolated from several studies of the general population suggest that males and non-whites experience the so-called "functional psychological disorders" less frequently but the neuropsychiatric disorders more frequently; data extracted from several studies of imprisoned offenders meet that expectation.

Indeed, consideration of epidemiological studies of mental health and disorder in the general population, inflected appropriately by the demographic characteristics that differentiate members of the incarcerated correctional population, leads quite clearly to the conclusion that the incidence of mental disorder in correctional populations is substantially confounded with the incidence of mental disorder in non-white, lower SES groups in the larger society.

It is reasonable for even the tough minded to speculate that, epidemiologically, the *rate* of serious mental disorder among members of correctional populations is at least as great as the median rate found in "fine screen" epidemiological studies of the general population — i.e., not lower than 19%.

But it is also reasonable to believe, on the basis of the reassembled Megargee-Bohn data, that methods of mental health census taking which mimic the professional diagnostic process (i.e., direct examination of subjects utilizing scientifically sound diagnostic instruments) rather than rely on the standard epidemiological technique (i.e., subject self-reports in response to an interview schedule administered by non-clinicians) are likely to yield mental disorder ratios in the correctional population dramatically higher than — and perhaps nearly four times as high as — that median figure.[14]

Even though significant mental retardation may constitute the grounds for exculpation, and one would therefore expect to find a virtually zero prevalence within the prison population, the extent of such retardation among prisoners exceeds that reported in epidemiological studies of the general population by a substantial margin.

Further, in view of the rather consistent finding of decisively higher levels of neuropsychiatric disorder among non-white groups and their over-representation in the correctional population, it is reasonable to believe that the disorders found among prisoners will be disproportionately more often those that directly involve or implicate neuropsychological or neurophysiological functioning.

Notes

1. "Psychosocial dysfunction" as operationally defined by Warheit, Bell, Schwab & Buhl (1986) appears to have much in common with the construct "social competence" advocated by Shah (1976) as preferable to the term "mental health" in application to a correctional population. In contrast to the diagnostic criteria for mental health and illness. Shall holds that social competence inheres in the capacity to select alternative behaviors to achieve goals, to utilize social systems and resources effectively, and to test reality effectively.

2. In his review of the research on coma and the etiology of violence, physician Carl Bell (1986) similarly concluded that, since "[Members of] lower socio-economic groups are more predisposed to brain injury from trauma" and in view of "the etiologic significance of central nervous system dysfunction in the production of violent behavior, physicians have a role in the early identification of potentially violent subjects." Bell associated head trauma leading to coma and resultant in largely undetected organic brain disorder both with race and with social class.

3. There is some reason to believe that, at least in some prisons in some states, a *majority* of inmates not only come from lower SES origins but indeed have been "state-raised" under the auspices of child protective agencies, which typically seek guardianship as a result of abuse or neglect. Children under

such protection, however, are usually shunted from one foster home to another; there are often feeble attempts at unwelcome outpatient psychotherapy along the way and/or periods of involuntary mental hospitalization as punctuation. In either case, it is indeed the situation that referral to mental health services has come through "court-related" channels, though not as a reult of criminal charges. Thus, in his study of the characteristics of inmates who aggress against other inmates (i.e., the "violent vs. the victimized," Wright (1991) observes: "Prison populations are composed of predominantly poor, lower-class segments of society who differentiate themselves along ethnic lines and are generally hostile to one another [a set of conditions that] promotes a climate which permits violence . . . in the explotive environment found in today's prisons, victims may simply be the unfortunate prey of exploitive state-raised convicts."

4.   Not surprisingly, the incidence of psychological research on those who commit criminal homicide substantially exceeds that devoted to those who commit offenses of other sorts. Some approximation to a mental health census among homicide offenders emerges from a number of studies.

Reports of the proportion of those convicted of murder (and thus excluding those accused but acquitted by reason of insanity) who exhibit clear symptoms of diagnosable psychiatric disorder range from a high of 100% to a low of 60%. In general, these studies are entirely *descriptive* rather than comparative — i.e., they do not essay to compare the rate of such disorder *either* between convicted murderers and those convicted of other crimes *or* between convicted murderers and the general population. The upper limit of 100% was reached in a study of convicted homicide offenders in the prisons of Finland by Keltikangas-Jarvinen (1978), with 71% of these diagnosed as psychopathically deviate, 21% as neurotic, and 7% as schizophrenic. Some 92% of similar offenders in the prisons of Scotland were diagnosed as dysthymic (depressed), neurotic, or delusional (Heather, 1977). Among murderers convicted in Contra Costa County, California, over a three-year period (Wilcox, 1985), 69% were diagnosed as psychotic (including those suffering from the drug-induced psychoses), brain-injured, addicted, or psychopathically deviate. In one study in Poland (Szymusik, 1972), 60%, and in another (Sila, 1977) 64%, of convicted murders were diagnosed as psychotic, alcohol-addicted, or suffering from degenerative brain disease. And, in a retrospective analysis of all known homicides in Iceland between 1900 and 1979, 66% of the offenders were post-diagnosed as psychotic, mentally retarded, neurotic, alcohol- or drug-dependent, or suffering from personality pattern disturbances (Petursonn & Gundjonsson, 1981).

Studies of convicted murderers are further amplified by reports on psychiatric disorder among those *accused* of homicide.

Thus, Daniel & Harris (1982) found "at least one primary psychiatric disorder," identified as schizophrenia, personality pattern disturbance, alcoholism, or organic psychosis, in 85% of the women charged with homicide who were examined at the University of Missouri College of Medicine. But these investigators found a *higher* rate of such disorder (93%) among the women they examined who were charged with crimes *other than* homicide.

In rather sharp contrast, Gillies (1976) reported that *no* psychiatric abnormality was found in 90% of the 367 men accused of murder in Glasgow between 1953 and 1974 who were examined at Stobhill General Hospital at the request of the prosecution. When the reciprocal rate of 10% of *accused* murderers with diagnosable psychiatric disorder in one large jurisdiction is juxtaposed to the 92% rate reported by Heather (1976) among *convicted* murderers in all of Scotland, the difference is no less than astounding.

Perhaps, however, some explanation is to be found in the speculations of Arboleda-Florez (1981) on the *post-homicidal induction of mental illness* immediately following arrest and while awaiting prosecution, in which the stressors associated with the experience of apprehension and detention are paramount. It may be arguable that the very high rates of diagnosable psychiatric disorder among convicted and imprisoned murderers reported in the several studies reviewed reflect disorders induced, or at least led from incipient to florid states, *following, and perhaps as a result of,* conviction and imprisonment.

These reports are augmented by a vast array of *clinical* case studies, usually of a single murderer, that amply demonstrate severe psychiatric disorder in the instant case, and by studies of those *acquitted* by reason of insanity, in which case severe mental disorder has been judicially determined. In virtually the only *comparative* study reported within a 15-year period, however, Langevin and his associates (1982) at Clarke Institute of Psychiatry, Toronto, compared the rates of psychiatric disorder observed among homicide offenders, offenders who had committed non-violent crimes, and a group of members of the community not accused or convicted of any crime, finding no significant differences in the rate of psychiatric disorder among or between the three groups.

The relevant studies, many of them undertaken outside the U.S., suggest an incidence of severe psychiatric disorder among convicted homicide offenders two to three times greater than that observed in epidemiological studies of the general population in this country and Canada. Because the diagnoses reflected in these studies were made after conviction, whether the disorders observed pre- existed the criminal act or whether they were induced after the commission of the crime, apprehension, prosecution, and, in most cases, imprisonment, must remain indeterminate.

Because the racial composition of the societies in which the majority of the relevant studies were undertaken differs from that of the U.S. in marked ways, conclusions emergent therefrom can be predicated of the U.S. only with extreme caution.

5. Indirectly, because their focal interests lay elsewhere (and perhaps inadvertently, since they did not reference the rich Megargee-Bohn literature), Bernstein & Garbin and their associates (1985, 1987) have provided data that corroborate the MMPI scale elevations reported in the principal Megargee-Bohn monograph. Bernstein & Garbin were interested in a factor analytic approach to simplifying the manifold dimensions of the instrument. In their research, they analyzed data first (1985) from a sample of 2000 Federal inmates and secondly from a sample of nearly 17,000 inmates (1987). The mean scale elevations they report on their inmate sample (1985, p. 777)

are highly congruent with those reported in the principal Megargee- Bohn source document.

6. Schuckit, Herrman & Schuckit (1977), however, estimated that only 5% of the offenders they examined required "acute treatment" of the character provided in a psychiatric hospital, while the remainder could be treated on site in the correctional facility, apparently through treatment modalities usually associated with outpatient mental health care.

7. Walters, White & Greene (1988) found serious mental disorder (that is, depression, mania, schizophrenia, schizophreniform disorder) on the basis of non-psychometric assessment through clinical review of case history and interview material among 78% of the inmates in a maximum security Federal prison. Their report contains sufficient detail to permit recalculation of mean values on MMPI scales for that portion of the sample found to be disordered on the basis of independent and non-psychometric clinical assessment; such recalculation indicates that the *mean* values for this group exceeded the threshold of clinical significance on the MMPI scales that measure paranoia and schizophrenia (as well as that which measures psychopathic deviation). Hence, the judgments reached on the basis of clinical, non-psychometric assessment are confirmed psychometrically on the MMPI.

   As if to provide cross-cultural, transnational validation not for the Megargee-Bohn methodology so much as for the relative incidence of disorder found in their original sample, Taylor (1986) reported that fully 66% of offenders sentenced to long terms in London displayed serious psychiatric disorder. Alternately, Washington & Diamond (1985) found serious psychiatric disorder in only 42% of the *women* inmates of five county jails in California. They opined, however, that community response both to mental disorder among women and to the incarceration of disordered women in correctional settings may have served to artificially deflate this ratio. Such considerations appear not to dissuade the decision to imprison women in Britain; instead, according to Carlen (1985), "Many women with previous histories of mental illness are sent to prison on the grounds that they are not [currently] mentally ill. Yet, once in prison, they are treated with massive doses of drugs on the grounds that they are mentally ill," as can be inferred from their histories. "The discipline settings of womens' prisons, far from engendering ordered states of mind, engender confused states of consciousness."

8. Substantial current research has been devoted to a phenomenon called "career criminality," with a general finding that formal criminal behavior (and particularly that reflected in crimes of violence) tends to decrease with age. In an impressive study (slightly flawed by reliance on data reflecting *arrests* rather than those reflecting *convictions)*, Blumstein & Cohen (1987) studied what they called the "criminal careers" of some 13,000 arrestees in Detroit and Washington, D.C., concluding that participation in crime tends to stabilize in early adulthood. At this point, many who commenced delinquent behavior in adolescence or earlier apparently forsake the criminal lifestyle, but those who do not apparently continue to commit crimes at a relatively constant rate for the remainder of their life-span. These data appear to support Blumstein & Moitra's (1980) earlier contention that a very small

proportion of persons (on the order of 6% of all those ever convicted) are responsible for a very large proportion (on the order of 52%) of all criminal activity. Buikhuisen's (1982) finding that, as a group, what he called "persistent" offenders tend to suffer more frequently from central nervous system dysfunctions implicated in learning, and therefore in impaired ability to profit from experience, may offer some explanation.

Particularly since scores on the *Pd* scale have rather consistently differentiated correctional populations from general populations, however, it may be germane to consider an "incidental" finding reported by Colligan, Osborne, Swenson & Offord (1988, p. 44) in the restandardization of the MMPI conducted at the Mayo Clinic, one major purpose of which was to produce contemporary norms inflected by both age and sex. Thus, these investigators reported that scores on the *Pd* scale were significantly negatively correlated with age among both male and female subjects in their restandardization sample (at r coefficients = -.30 and -.22, respectively); the same phenomenon was also observed on the scales that measure *paranoia* (at -. 19 and -.16), *mania* (at -.38 and -.25), and, among males only, *schizophrenia* (at -.20). These findings are remarkably congruent with the general direction of research in career criminality, so much so that one cannot help but wonder whether a naturally-occurring psychological phenomenon (which might, as Pallone & Tirman [1978] suggested, be termed "symptom abandonment" as a function of age) is not also reflected in decreases in overt criminal behavior.

More pertinently, Hare, McPherson & Forth (1988) analyzed the criminal careers over a 25 year period of Canadian offenders who had been identified in Hare's earlier studies as psychopaths or as non-psychopaths, reporting that "the criminal activities of non-psychopaths were relatively constant over the years, whereas those of psychopaths remained high until around age 40, after which they declined dramatically," adding that "The results are consistent with clinical impressions that some psychopaths tend to 'burn out' in middle age." Those clinical impressions are now psychometrically verified by the Mayo Clinic data base.

9. Lest the statistical purist blanch at these statements, one might hasten to add that the differences between proportions even in samples of quite discrepant size can be tested for significance through a variety of standard inferential techniques. Hence, if one calculates the Pearson chi square statistic with Yates' correction to test the significance of the differences in proportions with respect to each disorder represented in *Figure* 6, the resultant values reach incredibly high levels, ranging between 797 and 6066, with each statistically significant well beyond p = .0001; the exercise is another demonstration of the validity of Milton Rokeach's casual observation that, if one must calculate a test of significance to tell whether proportions are genuinely different, the data should probably be scrapped.

10. If one calculates the Yates-corrected chi square statistic to test the significance of the differences in proportions in *Figure* 7, the resultant value is 45.98 for the Denkowski & Denkowski proportion *vs.* the NIMH proportion, significant beyond p = .0001, but fails of significance at p = .01 for the Denkowski & Denkowski proportion *vs.* the Pasamanick proportion.

11. Current evidence appears to suggest that offenders sentenced to *probation* are less likely to recidivate than are those (likely, already "repeat") offenders sentenced to prison. Thus, in a discerning review of research data from four longitudinal studies of criminality, Petersilia (1980) concluded that only half of all those arrested once were ever arrested for a second offense; and, in a review of 55 studies of recidivism among 138 samples of parolees and 39 samples of probationers, Pitchard (1979) found that "auto theft is the only specific offense category consistently and significantly associated with recidivism."

Schneider, Schneider & Bazemore (1981) reported that only 9% of juvenile offenders remanded to a community services program rather than incarcerated had committed a subsequent offense; Roundtree, Edwards & Parker (1984) reported a recidivism rate of only 14% in their sample of 17- to 54-year-old probationers; and, in a study of releasees from a forensic psychiatric hospital ("for the criminally insane") in Canada, Pruesse & Quinsey (1977) found that only 46% of even this highly volatile and unpredictable group had recidivated during a four-year follow-up period. In contrast, in a follow-up study over a quarter century of the offense records of nearly 1600 subjects who had been convicted of violent crimes or of robbery in 1950, Miller, Dinitz & Conrad (1982) found a mean of nearly 8 rearrests, with half of these resulting in conviction; their data appear to support Blumstein & Moitra's (1980) contention that a very small proportion of offenders are responsible for a very large proportion of offenses. Whether these and similar data will also support the contention that prisons are themselves schools for the perfection of the skills required for future crime is another topic for another place. Given high rates of recidivism among *incarcerated* offenders and relatively low rates among offenders sanctioned by probation, it may be arguable that it is *simultaneously* the case that close to a majority of *convicted* felons do not recidivate and that the vast majority of *incarcerated* felons recidivate repeatedly (Buikhuisen & Meijs, 1983; Wormith & Goldstone, 1984).

12. It is highly probable that entry of a guilty plea represents not a decision of conscience on the part of the defendant but instead the result of plea-bargaining, a practice which to some major extent operationalizes the notion of "diminished responsibility" on a largely informal basis, often with minimal judicial oversight. In a plea-bargaining situation, an agreement is reached between the prosecutor and the defendant and his or her attorney that the charges on which the defendant has initially been indicted are to be reduced to charges (usually similar in character) that carry less severe sanctions. Though the rationale underlying the practice of plea-bargaining involves consideration of the costs associated with full-dress prosecution and jury trial as well as the complex issues associated with the development of convincing evidence and the credibility of witnesses, it is also reasonable to believe that some informal (and rather clearly extra-judicial) assessment of "extenuating circumstances" which diminish culpability or responsibility is among the variables considered by prosecutors in the decision whether to offer or to accept a bargained plea. As Berkley, Giles, Hackett & Kassoff (1977, p. 245) put it, 'The willingness of the prosecuting attorney to bargain in a particular case may be determined by the personal characteristics of the defendant — 'does he deserve a break'?"

Data reported in an earlier *Sourcebook* by Parisi, Gottfredson, Hindelang & Flanagan (1979, p. 545) from a major study of judicial practices in 1334 courts in 19 populous states indicate a *median rate of guilty pleas of 86% in all indictments for serious crime.* In the absence of comprehensive national data from all U.S. jurisdictions, there is no particularly strong reason to believe that this rate varies substantially, whether positively or negatively, in the courts and states not studied.

Data of national scope that speak to the extent to which the practice of plea-bargaining has preceded and produced so high a proportion of guilty pleas are not available. Indeed, empirical data on plea-bargaining have thus far been sparse and hardly revealing, a surprising state of affairs in view of what is assumed widely to be the universality of the practice. In some measure, the lack of responsive data may be explained by the finding that fully 69% of the criminal court judges responding to a nationwide survey of work styles in the courts reported that they were not aware of whether a plea bargain had been struck until the case actually came before them (Flanagan & McLeod, 1983, p. 110).

But, in the absence of firm data, we observe the opinion of Mr. Justice Peters of California in *In re Tahl* (1981 *California Reporter*, I California 3d, 140, p. 577) contemporaneously with the sentencing decisions reviewed in the RAND (Klein, Petersilia & Turner, 1990) study that: "A substantial portion — probably the vast majority — of criminal cases are disposed of through the process of plea-bargaining. We also know that most bargains do not appear on the record, and that defendants whose pleas have been obtained by promises of leniency are usually expected to deny the existence of such promises in spite of the common knowledge of judge, prosecutor, and defense counsel to the contrary. . . The result, in such cases, is that the entry of the plea is a ritual in which the recitations of the participants have little relation to reality."

The available data, then, indicate that a plea of guilty represents the *modal* manner of disposition in criminal cases; judicial opinion supports the inference that some very large proportion of those pleas result from bargaining. In these circumstances, final disposition of those cases in which a guilty plea is *not* entered is also of interest.

Once again, responsive data prove fragmentary and incomplete but instructive nonetheless. Data concerning the final disposition in all criminal cases in a given year in two rather dissimilar states, Florida and Connecticut, are reported by the U.S. Department of Justice's National Center for the State Courts (1979, pp. 67–70) in a study of the operation of those courts. In all criminal indictments in which a final disposition was reached in the year under study and in which a plea of guilty was *not* entered, conviction after trial occurred in 13.8% of the cases in Florida and in 8.5%. of the cases in Connecticut; conversely, charges were withdrawn or dismissed in 79% of the Florida cases and 86% of the Connecticut cases.

While extrapolations might prove interesting, the inescapable conclusions seem to be that the overwhelming majority of criminal convictions almost certainly issue from pleas of guilty, whether bargained or not, and that proceeding to trial is far more likely to produce withdrawal or dismissal of charges than any other result.

13. The conclusion of the RAND investigators, however, does not respond to other questions concerning race in the criminal justice system. For example, if the decision to offer a plea bargain in some measure pivots on the prosecutor's view that the defendant does or does not "deserve a break," as Berkley et al. have suggested, is that view itself influenced by racial factors, or perhaps by the confluence between race and "psychosocial dysfunction"?

14. By seeming to hold offenders to substantially higher standards for the identification of mental disorder than those utilized in epidemiological studies of mental health and illness in the general population or indeed than those used in clinical mental health practice, Monahan & Steadman (1982) reach quite different conclusions, a situation compounded by a rather uncritical adoption of their views by distinguished forensic psychiatrist Seymour Halleck (1987, pp. 2–3). Implicitly asserting that the standard methodologies in epidemiological studies tend to yield unrealistically high rates of mental illness, Monahan & Steadman make a distinction between "true" and "treated" cases of mental illness, observing that typically only 10% or so of the respondents in community surveys reported that they were "treated" (pp. 146–149); that distinction apparently ignores the fact that the major impetus for mental health census taking during the past quarter-century has been largely the need to establish public policy directions under the Federal Community Mental Health Act by inventorying the incidence of *untreated* cases. They also appear to wish to exclude from among those numbered as mentally ill all who are not severely psychotic (pp. 151, 165, 167), a limitation quite foreign either to epidemiological study or to clinical practice. Pursuing the distinction between "true" and "treated," Monahan & Steadman devote considerable attention to self-reported criminal behavior among former mental patients (pp. 155–164), an effort that will certainly illuminate the incidence of criminal behavior among those with verified mental disorder but *not* the incidence of mental disorder among those with verified criminal behavior.

   Moreover, in consequence of Hollingshead's (1986) observation that the criminal justice system itself represents the modal source of referral to treatment for members of the lowest SES group and the confounding of SES and race, especially when read in juxtaposition to data concerning characteristics of correctional populations, this approach appears to become quite circular. Further, at least among those persons suffering from those disorders in which *grandiosity* is a symptomatic characteristic (as in paranoid schizophrenia and certain other psychotic conditions), one might exercise extreme caution in accepting as accurate self-reports of criminal activity not concurrently confirmed by corroborating information.

   Even with these exclusions and limitations, however, when they turn to the obverse (i.e., the rate of mental disorder among those "known" to be criminal offenders), Monahan & Steadman (p. 153) adduce data from a study on the perceptions of arresting police officers *qua* clinical diagnosticians that indicate that these officers "diagnosed" 30% of their arrestees as mentally ill (18% as "somewhat" ill, 10% as "moderately" ill, 2% as "severely" ill, apparently quite apart from whether these arrestees were either independently or sequentially in toxic states of drug or alcohol use), nonetheless concluding that "If one assumes that police assessments . . . comport with psychiatric assessments (a major but not an unreasonable, assumption), these data are not inconsistent with those from community surveys of mental disorder" Indeed, the 30% rate precisely matches the median figure in the "gross screen" studies earlier reviewed and exceeds that in the "fine screen" studies by a ratio of 167%.

The general tenor of the Monahan & Steadman analysis appears to issue from an over-concern with whether a "causal" relationship obtains between mental disorder and criminal behavior (p. 182). If both criminal behavior and mental disorder are social deviancies, however, there need be no imputation either of causality or indeed even of relationship. In the clinical practice of medicine, few physicians would search, for example, for a relationship between athlete's foot and a broken arm in the same patient; instead, these "deviancies" from physical health would be construed as quite independent of each other and to be treated by quite independent therapeutic regimens.

3

Alcohol and Substance Abuse Disorders

The United States is a nation apparently obsessed by the use and abuse of chemical substances. In a typical year, the aggregate total of arrests made for offenses *exclusively* related to sale and possession of "controlled dangerous substances" (opium, cocaine, marijuana, or synthetics) *or* to alcohol (driving under the influence, public drunkenness, and other violations of liquor laws, such as sale to minors) and *not* related to felony crime exceeds the aggregate total of arrests made in all jurisdictions for *all* felony crimes *combined* (McGarrell & Flanagan, 1985, pp. 451–461) by a ratio of 175%.[1]

It may not be entirely coincidental that 40% of the specific pathological conditions, both "functional" and neuropsychiatric, cataloged in the *Diagnostic and Statistical Manual* of the American Psychiatric Association (1987) as constituting the universe of mental disorders are associated with the use or abuse of alcohol or other substances.

Such disorders cover a vast range, from essentially self-limiting conditions like intoxication through longer-term delirium or hallucinosis to relatively permanent neuropsychiatric conditions induced by the effects of particularly virulent substances on the biochemistry and even the morphology of the brain, which perpetuate as dementia, organic psychosis, or organic personality syndrome (Perry, 1987). With respect to alcohol and each class of "abusable substance," the associated psychological disorders include patterns of abuse, dependence syndromes, intoxication and withdrawal states, delusional disorders, and dementia.

Substance Abuse as Criminal and as Criminogenic

Offenses in which alcohol or drugs are implicated can be categorized as those which are legislatively defined as *criminal in themselves* (e.g., driving under the influence, possession of a controlled dangerous substance, whether for personal use or in sufficient quantity to suggest an intent to distribute) and those that are *criminogenic,* in the sense that alcohol or drugs contribute to felony offenses beyond the mere fact of substance misuse.

In a many jurisdictions, alcohol and drug offenses in the "criminal in themselves" category will, when not simultaneously linked to a felony crime independent of substance abuse charges, result in a relatively mild sanction — usually a fine or other penalty (e.g., suspension or revocation of a license to operate a motor vehicle) and placement on probation, perhaps with participation in a substance abuse rehabilitation program a requirement thereof. In these cases, the primary responsibility for behavior control and/or for engendering behavioral change is implicitly shifted from the correctional community to the mental health community. At least from the perspective of correctional management, offenders in this category are barely members of correctional populations.

Persons convicted of offenses in which alcohol or drug use has been criminogenic, however, will assuredly find their way into the correctional population, but the offenses-of-record in connection with their convictions will usually reflect only the felony offense in which alcohol or drugs have been criminogenic rather than the misuse of these substances themselves.

Engine, Lubricant, or Motive?

The use or abuse of alcohol and other psychoactive substances, whether "controlled" and "dangerous" or not and whether obtained illegally or through medical prescription, might be associated with felony crime in several ways:

- As *engine*, functioning so as to induce a person "under the influence" to commit a criminal act of which he/she might otherwise seem incapable when not actively intoxicated.
- As *lubricant*, functioning so as to facilitate what, at least *post-hoc*, appears to be a predisposition to criminal behavior, with the felony committed either "under the influence" or not.
- As *motive*, functioning as the goal to which criminal activity is directed, with the felony committed typically while the offender is *not* "under the influence."

The *engine* and *lubricant* functions correspond to what the late William McGlothlin (1985, p. 155) of UCLA has called the "direct pharmacological effects" of drug or alcohol use, among which he catalogs:

> drug-induced disinhibition resulting in impulsive actions, crimes of negligence such as those resulting from driver- impaired performance,

and the occasionally reported use of drugs . . . as a means of fortifying [oneself] to engage in criminal activities.

Biochemically-determined neuropsychological sequelae follow the use or abuse of psychoactive substances of various sorts. As cataloged in a variety of standard sources on psychopharmacology (Hofmann & Hofmann, 1975; Schatzberg & Cole, 1986; Frances & Franklin, 1988, pp. 313–355), each of the major classes of "abusable" substances possesses specific biochemical properties that produce predictable neuropsychological sequelae; these range from euphoria, aggressivity, and overwhelming impulsivity (as in the case of psychotomimetic central nervous system stimulants, such as cocaine and the amphetamines) through disinhibition of customary behavior control (alcohol) to persistent passivity and withdrawal (as in the case of narcoleptic central nervous system sedatives and depressants). It is likely that substances with variant biochemical properties may be *differentially* criminogenic in relation to criminal behavior of one sort, but not of other sorts — i.e., that the use or abuse of drugs with particular biochemical properties which produce predictable, but very particular, neuropsychological effects accelerates or contributes to particular types of criminal activity, but not to other types.

Hence, it is biochemically credible to suppose that the use or abuse of *central nervous system stimulants* (and perhaps of hallucinogens) accelerates *crimes of violence and personal victimization.* Among the property crimes, it seems likely that *burglary* alone might be accelerated by stimulants. Conversely, it is likely that the *central nervous system depressants retard violent behavior* of all sorts. These speculations, however, do not necessarily point to substance use or abuse as the primary *engine* for crime; instead, such use or abuse might more convincingly be regarded as a *lubricant* which potentiates other predisposing factors, both intra- and extra- personal. And almost certainly it is the *"profit crimes"* of burglary and robbery that are implicated when the acquisition of abusable substances functions as *motive.* In McGlothlin's (1985, pp. 154–155) formulation:

> drug use contributes to crime directly by potentiating impulsive and violent behavior . . . Alcohol is the only drug for which there is sufficient statistical data to establish a causal connection: the evidence clearly shows a relationship between acute effects and crimes of both violence and negligence . . . barbiturates have been found to

53

potentiate assaultiveness ... amphetamines and cocaine in high doses can produce paranoid reactions resulting in violence ... Marijuana and the stronger hallucinogens are also capable of producing psychotic reactions, and there are occasional references [in the research literature] to violent behavior during these episodes [but] marijuana typically decreases both expressed and experienced hostility ... there is growing evidence that the pseudohallucinogen, phencyclidine [i.e., PCP], has a fairly high potential for producing combative and violent behavior ... Opiates produce a reliable sedating reaction without the increased emotional lability and aggressiveness accompanying alcohol and barbiturate use. Thus, the pharmacological properties of opiates would be expected to decrease rather than potentiate criminal behavior, and this is generally consistent with the available evidence ... Finally, and perhaps this is the issue of major concern, there is the question of income-generating crime among individuals with expensive drug habits [and] commission of acquisitive crimes during a period of withdrawal.

Alcohol is something of a special case because of the paradoxical effects typically observed at low and at high levels of consumption. At high levels of consumption, alcohol produces the pattern of psychomotor retardation associated with central nervous system depressants. But at low levels of consumption (during what many experienced drinkers call the "rush" at first ingestion), alcohol produces what is commonly referred to as disinhibition of impulse control accompanied by a sense of exhilaration, a state of affairs conducive to aggressivity and assaultiveness (Frances & Franklin, 1987, pp. 141–143). Biochemically, it seems more likely that alcohol will prove criminogenic during the early or "rush" phases of ingestion than after prolonged ingestion. As Levin (1987, p. 19) has described the process:[2]

The sedative-hypnotics, including alcohol, initially depress the inhibitory synapses of the brain. Since the negation of a negative is a positive, the depression of the inhibitory synapses is excitatory. It is for this reason that alcohol is sometimes misclassified as a stimulant, although it is a depressant. Behaviorally, this disinhibition may manifest itself in high spirits and a devil-may-care attitude which may subjectively be experienced as euphoria. Anxiety is concomitantly reduced ... Excitatory synapses are soon also depressed, however, and the behavioral and experiential effects of alcohol catch up with its pharmacological effect, which has been depressive all along.

From the pioneering studies of premier criminologist Marvin Wolfgang (1958) onward, a considerable body of research evidence, much of it summarized by Collins (1981-*b)* and Roizen (1981), has pointed toward a consistent link between alcohol and violent crime; because of ubiquity and ease of access (at least since repeal of the Volstead Act), alcohol is apparently infrequently implicated as motive in profit crimes.

After reviewing the relevant studies, however, in a conclusion that precisely anticipated the findings of Langevin, Paitich, Orchard, et al. (1982) in their study of homicide offenders in Ontario over a decade, Blum (1981, pp. 115–116) proposed that the criminogenic character of alcohol consumption in relation to criminal violence is modulated by a number of impinging variables:

> Under no circumstances will alcohol be a sole "cause" of violence. Alcohol may alter perceptions, cognitive performance, moods/ emotions, and response capabilities and preferences. Less adaptive solutions, such as violence . . . occur with decrements in judgment. Violence may also be adaptive, or perceived as such . . . One expects that violence will occur when both preexisting and situational factors stimulate, facilitate, or permit it. Violence in association with alcohol may vary with dosage and, in turn, with pharmacologically specific effects including arousal levels, cognitive deficits and psychological reactions to such changes (e.g., anxiety).

"Tinder Box" Circumstance Leading to Violence

Blum's formulation is congruent with the view that criminal violence is more likely to occur under "tinder box" circumstances, in which the capacity to resolve either immediate or long-standing disputes by nonviolent means has been impaired by mood-altering substances. National data indicate, for example, that 60% of all criminal homicides occur under such "tinder box" circumstances.

Doubtless following Wolfgang & Ferracutti's (1967) characterization of an age-linked "subculture of violence," Wilson & Daly (1985) have interpreted "tinder box" circumstances as indicative of a "young male syndrome," in which "status competition, 'taste for risk,' dare-devilry and gambling" are said to be principal features. Observing that the data from some 700 homicides in Detroit indicate that "victim and offender populations were almost identical, with unemployed, unmarried young men greatly over-represented," these investigators propose that the "taste for risk" leading to homicide "is primarily a masculine attribute and is socially facilitated by the presence of peers in pursuit of the same goals."

In a study of violence among offenders and among former mental patients, Steadman (1982) confirmed that the presence of third parties in a conflict situation tends to potentiate the probability of violence. Felson & Steadman (1983) indeed identified what they described as a "systematic pattern" in tinder box homicides in a study of 159 such episodes:

> They began with identity attacks, followed by attempts and failures to influence the antagonists. Threats were made, and finally the verbal conflict ended in physical attack . . . retaliation is a key principle in the escalation of these incidents in that aggressive actions by the victim were associated with aggressive actions by the offender and the likelihood that the victim would be killed.

Luckenbill (1977) has termed this phenomenon a "character contest," in which the victim generally stipulates to violence as a means of conflict resolution. Strong empirical validation for the construct is found in a study by Fishbain, Fletcher, Aldrich & Davis (1987) which contrasted some 20 subjects who had died while playing Russian roulette with 95 who had committed suicide. The former were distinguished from the latter by a history of drug and alcohol abuse, and the investigators opined that they "were trying to treat their depression through risk taking behavior." Similarly, in a study that compared black women who committed homicide with their victims on a number of social characteristics, McClain (1982) concluded that the two groups "exhibit essentially similar behavior patterns that increase their probability of involvement in homicide," so that who becomes the victim and who the offender may be essentially a matter of the luck of the draw in a specific behavioral interaction.

Some support for the hypothesis that the person who emerges from the contest as victim has consented to violence in the resolution of conflict is found in a study by Budd (1982), of the Los Angeles Coroner's office, who reported that toxic levels of alcohol were found at autopsy in the blood samples of 61% of murder *victims*. The literary-minded will recall Stephen Crane's quatrain 'Two youth, in apparel that glittered," from *War Is Kind*, his 1897 collection of poetry, in which the self-identified victim, after proclaiming "I am glad to die thus, in this medieval fashion, according to the best legends . . . took the wound gladly, and died, smiling."

Clarke (1985) and other commentators have opined that such a "taste for risk" likely declines with advancing age; such an interpretation seems consistent with the findings of Loeber (1982), Holland & McGarvey (1984), and Blumstein & Cohen (1987) on the age-related decline in the emission of violent behavior. From an alternate perspective which does not, however, require the inferential invention of an internal trait/state like "taste for risk," it might be argued in respect of homicide that most males who are likely to kill have already done so by age 40 and, in consequence of the high ratio of apprehension and prosecution for homicide (in contrast to that for other felony crimes), are serving prison sentences thereafter; and all those "essentially similar" risk-takers who are likely to become victims are already dead.

"Pathological Intoxication" and Criminal Culpability

Delirium and dementia, whether induced by substance use or resultant from such other sources as cerebrovascular disease, are clinical conditions which seem clearly to impede knowing, informed, and voluntary behavior and thus would seem to constitute substantive evidence that a person who commits a criminal act while delirious or demented meets the stringent standards for exculpation embedded in the M'Naghten Rule. Promulgated in the decision of an English court in 1843 (and doubtless influenced by the views of Joseph Pritchard, an English physician who had earlier invented a mental illness he termed "moral insanity" [Pichot, 1978, p. 56] to explain criminal behavior), in a case in which the secretary to a cabinet officer was murdered by a disappointed office seeker who declared that he had been commanded by God to kill the Prime Minister, the M'Naghten Rule holds that legal culpability attaches to an otherwise criminal act only when the behaver knows in advance that the contemplated behavior counters moral principle and/or positive law.

As the editors of an important monograph commissioned by the Royal College of Psychiatrists (West & Walk, 1977, p. 1) put it: "If an offender knew that what he was doing was wrong, he was legally sane and subject to punishment." Thus, under the M'Naghten formulation, a person who is incapable of distinguishing "wrong" from "right" is *not* to be held legally culpable.

On this side of the Atlantic, two cases in the last quarter of the last century (*Parsons v. the State of Alabama,* adjudicated in 1887, and *Davis v. United States,* adjudicated a decade later) added the "irresistible impulse" test, which exculpates a person who is incapable of resisting an impulse propelling him or her to a wrong or legally criminal act (Stone, 1976, p. 229), i.e., when he or she is *not* "free to choose" whether to behave or not in response to a stimulus situation.

In 1954, the U.S. District Court for the District of Columbia specifically included prior mental illness in the catalog of acceptable justifications for a claim of non-culpability under M'Naghten by holding that "an accused is not criminally responsible if his unlawful act was the product of mental disease." Following the name of the defendant (Durham) and the presiding justice (Bazelon) in the case, the resultant principle is called the *Durham Test* or the *Bazelon Rule*.

Over the course of nearly a century and a half, a variety of other justifications have been accepted by the courts under M'Naghten to explain either the incapacity to distinguish right from wrong or the incapacity to resist the impulse to behave criminally (Rogers, 1986, pp. 39–90). Hence, in its model penal code, the American Law Institute proposed a more comprehensive statement (Stone, 1976, p. 230):

> A person is not responsible for criminal conduct if, at the time of such conduct, as a result of mental disease or defect he lacks substantial capacity either to appreciate the criminality of his conduct or to conform his conduct to the requirement of law. [But] the terms "mental disease or defect" do not include an abnormality manifested only by repeated criminal or otherwise antisocial conduct.[3]

In its 1982 statement on the insanity defense, however, the American Psychiatric Association (1984, p. 17) essentially endorsed a modification of the American Law Institute standard for insanity (and, by extension, for diminished criminal responsibility) set forth by University of Virginia professor of law R.J. Bonnie that excludes the "voluntary ingestion of alcohol or other psychoactive substances" as an acceptable argument for exculpation. Bonnie's formulation, with added emphases:

> A person charged with a criminal offense should not be found guilty by reason of insanity if it is shown that as a result of mental disease or mental retardation he was unable to appreciate the wrongfulness of his conduct at the time of the offense. As used in this standard, the terms mental disease or mental retardation include only those severely abnormal mental conditions that grossly and demonstrably impair a person's perception or understanding of reality *and that are not attributable primarily to the voluntary ingestion of alcohol or other psychoactive substances.*

After publication of the Association's statement, a number of legislatures adopted what are called "pathological intoxication" laws that directly incorporate either the Bonnie formulation or a close analogue thereto. In some states, the legislation contains a provision concerning the "novelty" of the substance ingested by a particular accused offender, to the effect that a defendant who has never ingested a particular substance before, and therefore cannot reasonably be expected to have anticipated its effects, may still invoke in his or her defense a claim of involition or lack of knowledge in respect of a subsequent criminal act.

Overall, the impact of the Association's amendment and its incorporation into law has been to remove substance-induced intoxication, delirium, and dementia from the arena of mental disorder and to situate them in the arena of "willful misconduct," a position apparently supported by the Supreme Court of the United States in its decision in *Traynor v. Turnage,* 1988.[4] The implicit conclusion would seem to be that these substance-induced states not only do not serve to exculpate, but may even serve to further *inculpate* the offender.

Indeed, the tendency toward increased inculpation may operate at a very elemental level. There is at least impressionistic evidence that scene-of-the-crime arrest (rather than an on-scene intervention short of arrest) is more likely when the putative offender, but not the victim, is perceived by police to be under the influence of alcohol (Greenberg, 1981, p. 93). That effect is apparently compounded by socioeconomic status and, since race is confounded with SES, perhaps by race as well. In their review of drinking patterns inflected by SES, Polich & Kaelber (1985, p. 62) conclude: "Those with low economic and social status are less likely than others to drink, but more likely to get into trouble if they drink." About other formal mental disorders, like dependence syndromes and the perpetuation of substance abuse as organic psychoses or organic personality disorders, the law has thus far been silent.

Nonetheless, the inconsistency implicit between the APA's position and the fact that not less than 15% of the total of the 374 text pages in its 1987 revision of the *Diagnostic and Statistical Manual of Mental Disorders* is devoted to a cataloging of the wide panoply of alcohol and substance abuse syndromes, ranging from dependence to intoxication and delirium — with the latter two surely indicative of a state of mind that is, by the APA's own definitions, hardly congruent with unimpaired "perception or understanding of reality," let alone appreciation of the wrongfulness of one's conduct — glows with crystalline clarity.

Incidence of Alcohol and Substance Abuse

Intoxication and habituation to mood-altering substances of a variety of sorts (not limited to alcohol and those illicit drugs that have been legislatively declared "controlled dangerous substances," but including medicants available by prescription as well) biochemically trigger psychological states that are relatively substance-specific, each with predictable behavioral consequences. Among the most troublesome of these states (associated with some abusable substances, but not with others) are aggressivity and impulsivity, which often find expression in behavior that is formally criminal. It should not be surprising, then, to find a high incidence of substance abuse disorders in correctional populations.

Variant Methods of Inquiry

Early studies of the relationship between substance use or abuse and felony crime prototypically relied on data from self-reports, often of the offender but sometimes of the victim, as the standard index of criminogenic substance use or abuse, with but few inquiries relying on independent observations and yet fewer based on laboratory assessments of whether alcohol or drugs (licit or illicit) could be detected in the physical system of an accused (or witnessed) offender. Independent observations (most often by arresting police officers, or, far less frequently, by a knowledgeable witness) varied, but essentially only marginally, from self-reports of victim or offender.

Contemporary studies of the relationship between substance use or abuse and felony crime can be categorized by method of inquiry into those which utilize *self-report* data and those which employ *laboratory assay methods.* Among the self-report studies, there is a further distinction between those investigations that inquire into the alcohol and/or substance use or abuse habits of *known offenders* and those that inquire into the *criminal behavior patterns of known alcohol or substance users.*

Among the laboratory assay studies, there is also a further distinction, predicated on the "sensitivity" of the specific methodology (Wish, 1990) used to detect metabolites which biochemically succeed the ingestion of "controlled dangerous substances" or to determine blood alcohol content, typically among samples of arrestees, and even then, given the relative infrequency of instant apprehension, often long after the criminal event. From the perspective of criminogenesis though not particularly from that of correctional management, to interpret appropriately studies utilizing either laboratory assay or self-report methods, it is often necessary to regroup the data reported so as to eliminate those cases in which the offenses-of-record are related exclusively to substance abuse or alcohol laws.

Criminal Behavior Among Known Substance Abusers

A number of investigations, both in this country (Newcomb & Bentler, 1988; Nurco, Ball, Shaffer & Hanlon, 1985; Nurco, Shaffer, Ball & Kinlock, 1984), in Britain (Gordon, 1983; Hammersley & Morrison, 1987, 1988), and in Sweden (Fry, 1985; Torstensson, 1987) have addressed criminal activity among known substance abusers. In some cases, data were collected from retrospective interviews with persons currently identified as drug or alcohol abusers (Ball & Nurco, 1984; Hunt, Lipton & Spunt, 1984; Inciardi, Pottieger & Faupel, 1982; Tuchfeld, Clayton & Logan, 1982); in others, more elaborate research designs collected longitudinal data on subjects who had applied for (and/or completed) treatment in drug rehabilitation facilities operated by mental health authorities (Martin, Cloninger & Guze, 1982; Rosenthal & Nakkash, 1982).

Some studies, particularly those which relied on the retrospective self-reports of known abusers, produced such astounding data — e.g., Ball, Rosen, Flueck & Nurco (1982) report that their sample of 243 subjects had been responsible for 473,000 serious felony crimes over a period of eleven years, or 1946 crimes per person, or one crime every two days — that distinguished criminologist James Inciardi (1982) was led to severe criticisms of certain research designs as likely conducive to eliciting fraudulent data.

Among the most carefully designed and executed investigations, McGlothlin's (1985) is a prime exemplar. His subjects were 581 self-identified male narcotics addicts (mean age = 25; no racial data supplied) admitted to a treatment program in California who were followed over a ten year period after admission through periodic interviews *and* collection of police arrest records. Data concerning arrests for drug and other offenses, extent of drug dealing activity, employment, number of crimes self-reported annually, the number of person-days per year during which each subject self-reported as engaged in criminal activity, and a variety of other variables were arrayed in several ways. Of the several arrays, the most pertinent is that which contrasts subjects who used narcotics on a daily basis (and could thus be classified according to any lexical scheme as "addicts") with those who used narcotics less frequently.

In this contrast, the addicts were arrested significantly more frequently each year for *felony property offenses* and for *drug offenses*, but not for violent felonies; more frequently self-reported as engaged in drug dealing (58% vs. 16%); and self- reported a significantly higher number of *property* crimes per year (47 vs. 17), a higher level of income from crime ($9100 vs. $1700), and a significantly smaller proportion of person-days per year during which they were *not* engaged in criminal activity (53% vs. 83%).

Considering his own data and data from some 45 other studies that investigated the criminal behavior of *known* drug abusers over long periods of time, McGlothlin (1985, pp. 166–167) reached what he called "unequivocal conclusions" that "during periods of addiction, individuals are more likely to be arrested . . . to commit more crime, and to acquire more money from property crimes." Since the crimes committed by these known-addict subjects are predominantly property crimes (with the crimes of violence observed virtually invariably themselves associated with "drug deals gone sour"), McGlothlin's results seem to argue that, for abusers of one class of controlled dangerous substance, drug use functions criminogenically primarily as *motive*.

Curiously, despite the substantially greater period of time during which careful scientific study of the behavioral effects of alcohol use has progressed, few studies of known alcoholics (or "problem drinkers") have reached the clarity and precision of McGlothlin's among drug abusers. Perhaps the ubiquity and ease of legal access to alcohol have encouraged fewer of those who overuse this substance to seek treatment than those whose use of other substances *de facto* violates the law[5] and for whom participation in community-based treatment may even represent an alternative to prosecution. The stringent confidentiality maintained by Alcoholics Anonymous, without question the principal source of treatment nationwide and worldwide, may further discourage detailed investigation.

Hence, in his summary of the studies relevant to criminal behavior among known alcoholics, Collins (1981-*a*, pp. 164–166) cites data that suggest that only between 3% and 10% of self-identified "problem drinkers" arrayed by age in five-year intervals between 21 and 59 reported "police problems" during the immediately preceding thirty-six months. But the character of these problems is not specified and may range the spectrum from warnings for boisterousness through traffic charges to arrest (or conviction) for violent felony. Rather discrepant data are cited by Greenberg (1981) in her review of studies of alcoholics admitted voluntarily for inpatient or outpatient treatment, in which 11.5% appears as the median rate for the proportion of subjects in these groups who self-reported that they had been arrested *or* convicted for a criminal offense *not* related to alcohol use.

Substance Abuse among Offenders

In contrast to the lack of enumerative data in respect of general mental health, several major studies of inmates of jails and prisons have been completed by the U.S. Bureau of the Census for the Bureau of Justice Statistics, based on interviews with inmates conducted according to standard schedules by trained Census interviewers.

One such inquiry surveyed a stratified sample of 6000 inmates of jail facilities (Bureau of Justice Statistics, 1980) carefully chosen to accurately represent the parent population approximating 160,000. In the parent population, some 91,500 (94% male, 57% white), or 57% of all inmates, had been *convicted* of felonies (29.5%) and were awaiting incarceration in a state prison *or* of misdemeanors of various sorts (70.5%) and serving their sentences in these jail facilities. Self-reports were obtained concerning both alcohol consumption prior to the offense-of-record and the judgments of these subjects concerning whether they were "under the influence" of controlled dangerous substances at the time of the offense. The relevant data (*Ibid.*, p. 17) are recapitulated in *Figure* 9.

According to their self-reports, 51% of the subjects in this largely misdemeanant pool had, prior to the instant offense, consumed

Figure 9. Self-Assessed Alcohol and Drug Use Prior to the Offense of Record among Convicted Offenders Serving Sentences in Jail Facilities (Bureau of Justice Statistics, 1980).

Alcohol consumption prior to instant offense	
Had not consumed alcohol	51%
Had consumed less than 4 ounces	16%
Had consumed more than 4 ounces	28%
Had consumed an unknown quantity	2%
Consumption level not recorded	3%
Self-assessment of influence of drugs during instant offense	
Not under the influence of drugs	75%
Under the influence of drugs	21%
Heroin only	4%
Marijuana only	7%
Other drugs only	5%
Multiple drugs	5%
Drug influence not recorded	4%

alcohol, with 28% reporting that they had consumed in excess of four ounces. In addition, some 22% reported that they were, at the time of the instant offense, "under the influence of drugs." There is no reliable indication as to whether such "influence" at the time of the instant offense represented a continuing pattern of use or abuse among these *convicted* offenders, nor whether chronic use or abuse had additionally engendered identifiable psychological, psychophysiological, or neuro-psychiatric disorders. However, in the same survey, some 68% of all inmates (whether convicted or awaiting trial) admitted to drug use at some point in their lives, and nearly 40% admitted to daily use at some point in their lives (*Ibid.*, p. 16).

In a similar survey by the U.S. Bureau of the Census among convicted felons incarcerated in state prisons (Bureau of Justice Statistics, 1988), interviews were conducted with a stratified sample of 12,000 inmates (96% male; 49.7% white) carefully selected to represent accurately the total population of nearly 500,000 prisoners. Some 55% of the sample (and the parent population) had been convicted of crimes of violence (homicide, kidnapping, rape, sexual assault, robbery, assault), 31% of property offenses (burglary, larceny or theft, arson, fraud), 6% of drug offenses (possession, trafficking), and 4% of "public order" offenses (weapons possession, prostitution, and violation of probation or parole). Data on subjects' self-assessment of whether they were under the influence of alcohol or drugs at the time of the instant offense (*Ibid.*, p. 6) are recapitulated in *Figure* 10.

The final set of figures in *Figure* 10 suggests that very high pro-portions of offenders perceived themselves to have been under the influence of some mood-altering substance, or some combination of substances, during the offense for which they were currently incar-cerated. These self-report data are largely consistent with the body of data drawn from such smaller scale studies as those of Holcomb & Adams (1985) and Welte & Miller (1987) on incarcerated violent and non-violent offenders and further accord with the observations of Lewis, Cloninger & Pais (1983) and Tuchfeld, Clayton & Logan (1982) on the interactive relationship between alcohol use, substance abuse, and felony crime.

Laboratory Studies of Arrestees

Additional data on drug use or abuse among putative offenders are found in studies of *arrestees* which have utilized sophisticated labora-tory assays to detect the metabolites of a variety of controlled dangerous

Figure 10. Self-Assessed Alcohol and Drug Use Prior to the Offense of Record among Convicted Offenders Serving Sentences in State Prisons (Bureau of Justice Statistics, 1988).

Under the influence of alcohol during instant offense

Crimes of violence	20%
Property crimes	18%
Drug offenses	6%
Public order offenses	28%
All other offenses	12%
All offenses combined	19%

Under the influence of drugs during instant offense

Crimes of violence	13%
Property crimes	21%
Drug offenses	32%
Public order offenses	13%
All other offenses	13%
All offenses combined	17%

Under the influence of both alcohol and drugs during instant offense

Crimes of violence	20%
Property crimes	18%
Drug offenses	11%
Public order offenses	12%
All other offenses	14%
All offenses combined	18%

Under the influence of either or both alcohol and/or drugs during instant offense

Crimes of violence	54%
Property crimes	57%
Drug offenses	48%
Public order offenses	53%
All other offenses	39%
All offenses combined	54%

substances at, or soon after, the point of apprehension, whether under "hot pursuit" or other circumstances. In contrast to the Census surveys of probability samples representative of the national population of convicted offenders, these costly and labor-intensive laboratory assays have been limited to arrestees in particular jurisdictions (Graham, 1990).

Thus, Wish, Brady & Cuadrado (1986) studied arrestees in New York County, New York (Manhattan). Urine specimens for 5571 arrestees (97% male; 84% of all those arrested for felony or misdemeanor during a seven-month period; no racial data indicated) for the presence of four substances (cocaine, methadone, morphine, and phencyclidine or PCP) through "enzyme multiplied immune urine test" (EMIT) technique, a laboratory methodology described as 50% to 100% "more sensitive for identifying recent drug use" than other laboratory methods.[6] Specimens were collected at a central booking location before subjects were sent to court for arraignment. With those arrested for misdemeanors and/ or for drug or alcohol offenses only excluded, the reassembled data indicate that, when arrestees for suspected felony offenses (64% of all arrestees) are arrayed by type of offense charged, the "positive" rates found by laboratory analysis are remarkably high, generally exceeding those found by self-report inquiry among convicted felons by at least 100%, with 53% of those arrested for crimes of violence and 57% of those arrested for property crimes drug positive.

EMIT laboratory methodology was also utilized in a study of arrestees in the District of Columbia by Toborg & Bellassai (1987), who examined the urine specimens for 6160 arrestees (82% male; apparently an indeterminate proportion of all those arrested for felony or misdemeanor between June 1984 and January 1985; 83% black; 34% charged with misdemeanors only; 41% with prior convictions for either felony or misdemeanor) for the presence of amphetamines, cocaine, heroin, methadone, and phencyclidine (PCP). In this investigation (again, with arrestees for misdemeanors and for substance use charges excluded), the drug positive rate was 41% for arrestees for crimes of violence and 45% for arrestees for property crimes. The relevant (and reassembled) data from these investigations are recapitulated in *Figure* 11.[7]

Wish & O'Neil (1989) have consolidated data from the National Institute of Justice's "drug use forecasting" studies in 13 cities, through which "voluntary and anonymous" urine specimens of samples of arrestees were analyzed through EMIT technology for the metabolites of eight controlled dangerous drugs and two pharmacological preparations (Darvon, Valium) that have become subject to abuse. Among

Figure 11. Drug-Positive Rates among Arrestees for Felony Crime Based on Laboratory Assay Methods.

Among arrestees for crimes of violence	
Toborg & Bellassai, 1987	41%
Wish, Brady & Cuadrado, 1986	53%
Among arrestees for property crimes	
Toborg & Bellassai, 1987	45%
Wish, Brady & Cuadrado, 1986	57%

male arrestees, the proportions found drug-positive range from 50% in Indianapolis to 85% in San Diego; among females, the proportions range from 44% in Dallas to 87% in the District of Columbia. The presentation of source data in the Wish & O'Neil report does not permit segregation of arrestees for felony crime from those arrested for other offenses (including drug offenses), nor arraying drug positive rates by offense charge.

How Discrepant Are the Discrepancies?

What appear to be discrepancies of some considerable magnitude (which may be more important for those interested in the construction of a theory of criminogenesis than for those charged with the operation of correctional facilities, however) emerge from contrasts between data from the Census studies, based on self-reports of convicted inmates of jails and prisons, and laboratory assay data from studies of arrestees. Data from the laboratory studies suggest that nearly two of every five (Toborg & Bellassai) or one of every two (Wish, Brady & Cuadrado) accused offenders admitted to a jail facility immediately after arrest for a serious felony charge are actively "under the influence," a level of *drug* use (apart from alcohol use) that exceeds the level self-reported by convicted offenders by ratios of 200% to 300%. However unsatisfactory the research picture may be from the perspective of the theory of criminogenesis,[8] the implications in the practical order for management, security, and programming in correctional facilities and perhaps including provision for detoxification in jail facilities, are dramatic.

One might look to systematic differences in various jurisdictions relating to arrest and to the progression from arrest to conviction and incarceration to reconcile these discrepancies; and here jurisdictional particularities may well have a profound role. Given markedly low rates of indictment and conviction following arrest, is there any particularly sound reason to believe that more than a minor portion of the arrestees represented in these samples will later be incarcerated? What proportion of actively-toxic, readily-identifiable felony arrestees might reasonably be expected to find their way into a Treatment Alternative to Street Crime (TASC) substance abuse program, or a variant pretrial intervention alternative? In what proportion of the cases might the abuse of drugs itself constitute the grounds for a "diminished responsibility" pleading[9] that results in placement on probation, especially in the case of a first, non-violent felony offense? Some combination of such local jurisdictional factors might well reconcile the wide discrepancies observed between self-report data and laboratory data.

Base Rates in the General Population

Widely quoted data on the per capita consumption of alcohol per annum among the general population fail to reflect either pathological consumptive habits or the psychological or neuro-psychiatric effects thereof.

In an extensive review of the survey research conducted with stratified samples representative of the adult population of the nation (and relying on self-reports supplied by respondents), Polich & Kaelber (1985, p. 61) concluded that 75% of the adult men and 60% of the adult women in the nation consume beverage alcohol. Of these, a "high level of alcohol-related problems" (i.e., adverse psychosocial consequences) is found among 15% of the male consumers and 4% of the female consumers. Kolb & Gunderson (1985) estimate that approximately 20% of alcohol users can be expected to develop other serious *mental* disorders concomitantly with, or as the result of, such use.

On the basis of the Polich & Kaelber figures, a *base rate for psychosocial problems associated with alcohol use* among the general population can be calculated by syllabicating proportions. Thus, the base rate is projected at 11.25% (i.e., 15% of the 75% of adult males who use alcohol) among men and at 2.4% (4% of the 60% of adult females who use alcohol) among women. If one applies the estimates of Kolb & Gunderson (1985), the base rate among men would be calculated at 15% (i.e., 20% of 75%) and among women at 12% (i.e., 20% of 60%). On the basis of similar calculations, Hartman (1988, p. 160) estimates that there are nine million "problem drinkers" in the United States.

The proportions that result from these calculations, however, substantially exceed that in the National Institute of Mental Health Epidemiological Catchment Area studies, in which Burke & Regier (1988, p. 82) reported that 4.7% of the nearly 19,000 subjects surveyed by means of the NIMH Diagnostic Interview Schedule were categorized as suffering from "alcohol abuse/dependence" disorders.

The consumption of controlled dangerous substances itself constitutes criminal behavior, so that self-reports of the use of such substances itself constitutes an admission of illegality (Burke & Regier, 1988, p. 88).

Nonetheless, the most recent *National Household Survey on Drug Abuse* conducted by the National Institute on Drug Abuse (1987, pp. 10–25, 30–33, 46–49), based on a stratified sample of house-holds representative of those in the nation, reports that 33% of respondents over the age of 12 admitted to the use of marijuana at least once in their lives, 12% to the use of cocaine, 7% to the use of hallucinogens, and 9% to the use of stimulants (and 86% to the use of alcohol), with these categories not mutually exclusive.

There is no strong basis for an estimate regarding perpetuation of drug use (or, in the case of these surveys, perhaps only "experimentation") into serious drug-induced mental disorders, but, if anything, the effects of psychotomimetic substances like cocaine on brain functioning are physically more devastating than those of alcohol.

In a review of the relatively small number of studies that have followed longitudinally subjects who reported use of controlled dangerous substances at least once, Croughan (1985, p. 97) reports that "dependence" followed such use at ratios ranging from 2% to 10%. If we apply the higher ratio reported by Croughan to the proportion of the population that admitted to ever having used marijuana, the most frequently used of the several substances covered in the NIDA

Figure 12. Relative Frequency with Which Substance Use/Abuse Disorders Were Observed among Respondents in the NIMH Epidemiological Catchment Studies (Burke & Regier,1988) and among Prisoners in Bureau of the Census Studies (1988).

Disorder	Prisoners	NIMH Subjects
Alcohol use/dependence	*19%*	*4.7%*
Drug use/dependence	*17%*	*2.0%*
All substance use/abuse combined	*54%*	*6.0%*

survey (and, in the process, make the questionable assumption that equally serious sequelae follow experimentation with any controlled dangerous substance, regardless of biochemistry), one projects that, at most, the incidence of drug-induced mental disorders in the general population is 3%. That proportion is very close to the figure in the National Institute of Mental Health Epidemiological Catchment Area studies, in which Burke & Regier (1988, p. 82) reported that some 2% were categorized as suffering "drug abuse/dependence" disorders. Data from the NIMH studies on the general population and from the Bureau of the Census study on prisoners are recapitulated in *Figure* 12.[10]

Conclusion

In studies of the epidemiology of drug and alcohol use in the general population, mere "involvement" with the police or the courts on whatever charge (including possession of controlled dangerous substances, driving while intoxicated, etc.) is held to be indicative of "serious" problems associated with substance use. By that standard, commission of a crime (no less than apprehension and prosecution therefor) *not* associated with substance use while "under the influence" is most assuredly indicative of "serious" problems consequent to such use.

According to extrapolations from national data concerning alcohol consumption and the likelihood of serious problems attendant thereupon, the incidence of serious problems attendant upon alcohol consumption can be expected to vary among males in the range between 11.25% and 15%. Applying the same standard to correctional populations, *Census data [Figure 9] suggest an incidence among convicted offenders between three and four times that to be expected in the general population.*

According to extrapolations from national data concerning drug use and the likelihood of serious problems consequent thereto, the incidence of consequent serious problems can be expected to approximate 3%. Applying the same standard to correctional populations, *Census data suggest an incidence among convicted offenders between seven and twelve times that to be expected in the general population* and *laboratory assay studies [Figure 10] suggest an incidence among felony arrestees between fifteen and twenty times greater than that found in the general population.*

According to extrapolation from data in the NIMH Catchment Area studies [*Figure* 6], *Census data suggest an incidence of alcohol problems among prisoners eight times as great as that found in the general population and of drug use problems nineteen times as great as in the general population.*

Notes

1. Of all arrests (some 12,000,000) in all jurisdictions in the U.S. for all offenses (whether felony or misdemeanor), some 449,000 are made for violent felonies and some 1,930,000 for property felonies, while some 3,500,000 arrests are made *exclusively* for alcohol offenses and some 662,00 *exclusively* for drug offenses *not* associated with those felony crimes enumerated in the U.S. Department of Justice's Index of Serious Crime (i.e., homicide, assault, rape, robbery, weapons possession, burglary, forgery or fraud, larceny).

2. An alternate explanation incorporates hypoglycemia (a rapid decrease in blood glucose level) as a modulator in the link between alcohol and violence. As Pernanen (1981, p. 19) puts it: "Hypoglycemia has been [reported] as a factor responsible for violent behavior. Alcohol is known to cause hypoglycemia in individuals who are under-nourished. Since much excessive alcohol use is associated with poor nutritional habits, this condition could be a factor in explaining the association between prolonged alcohol use and violent crime." According to Berkow & Fletcher (1987, p. 1084), alcohol-induced hypoglycemia results both from nutritional deficiency and impairment in the capacity of the liver to metabolize glucose, with the impairment itself perhaps due to heavy alcohol usage (p. 870).

3. The final exclusion in the ALI standard — viz., that "the terms 'mental disease or defect' do not include an abnormality manifested only by repeated criminal or otherwise antisocial conduct" — would seem to preclude a diagnosis of *psychopathic deviation* (or, in the American Psychiatric Association's current lexicon, antisocial personality disorder) as an acceptable basis for an insanity defense. While the APA's (1984) formal modification as quoted *supra* contains no such exclusion, its Statement on the Insanity Defense elsewhere makes its "legislative intent" quite clear: "Allowing insanity acquittals in cases involving persons who manifest primarily 'personality disorder' such as antisocial personality disorder (sociopathy) does not accord with . . . psychiatric beliefs concerning the extent to which such persons do have control over their behavior. Persons with antisocial personality disorders should, at least for heuristic reasons, be held accountable for their behavior. The American Psychiatric Association, therefore, suggests that any revision of the insanity defense standards should indicate that mental disorders potentially leading to exculpation must be *serious.* Such disorders should usually be of the severity (if not always of the quality) of conditions that psychiatrists diagnose as psychoses" (p. 17).

    Those are stern words indeed, especially when juxtaposed with the description of antisocial personality disorder which the Association (1987, pp. 342–343) promulgates in its *Diagnostic and Statistical Manual of Mental Disorders:* "The disorder is often extremely incapacitating . . . Predisposing factors are Attention Deficit Hyperactivity Disorders . . . during prepuberty . . . Other predisposing factors include abuse as a child . . . Psychoactive Substance Abuse Disorders are commonly associated diagnoses . . . The disorder is more common in lower-class populations [and] People with this disorder are more likely than people in the general population to die prematurely by violent means." The decision rule to be followed in differential diagnosis reeks of Wonderland (p. 344): "*Schizophrenia* may present with some of the features of Antisocial Personality Disorder, such as impairment in occupational functioning and parenting; but the additional diagnosis of Antisocial Personality Disorder should be made only if there is a clear pattern of antisocial behavior."

The inconsistency between (*a*) a description of an "extremely incapacitating" mental disorder that results from "abuse as a child," is "more common in lower-class populations," and can be differentiated from schizophrenia only by a set of mental gymnastics that would do the Mad Hatter proud and (*b*) the judgment that those who suffer this disorder "should, at least for heuristic reasons, be held accountable for their behavior" can hardly be described as less than staggering — and perhaps even as indicative that the seductiveness of the "blame the victim" mind-set has become boundlessly pervasive.

4.   *Traynor v. Turnage* concerned a situation in which the Veterans Administration had denied continuation of GI Bill educational benefits to two veterans (Eugene Traynor and James P. McKelvey) who had developed a habit not uncommon among college students. Though they registered for a full program of courses each semester, they withdrew from their registered courses — as a result, they claimed, of excessive alcohol consumption; in other words, they got drunk too often to be attentive to class requirements.

The Veterans Administration's guidelines limit receipt of GI Bill educational benefits to a certain number of semesters, during which the recipient is expected to be in active pursuit of an academic program unless precluded by illness. Since the Federal Congress had, through its amendments to the Vocational Rehabilitation Act in the mid-1970s, seemed to have legislatively defined alcoholism as a disease, each veteran claimed that his withdrawal was predicated upon sound medical reasons.

The Veterans Administration took the opposite position, countering in essence that the alcoholism of these two veterans was the effect of "voluntary misbehavior" and thus terminated payment of benefits. In a set of legal proceedings that consumed several years, the U.S. Supreme Court upheld the Veterans Administration's decision — amid a substantial outcry both among members of the scientific community, among members of the general public interested in the control and treatment of alcoholism, and, not incidentally, among some members of the Congress. There the matter stood, however, until the final days of the Reagan Administration, when the retiring Congress in essence obviated the effect of the Supreme Court's decision by adopting Public Law S. 2049, which specifically directed the Veterans Administration to allow alcoholic veterans who could demonstrate a good faith effort to remedy their condition (e.g., by participating in a rehabilitation program) to apply for an extension of benefits on that account.

In the academic world, philosopher Herbert Fingarette (1988, 1990) of the University of California at Santa Barbara is the leading spokesperson for the "willful misconduct" perspective on alcoholism.

As Fingarette (1990, p. 6) sees it: "When behavior is labeled a disease, it becomes excusable because it is regarded as involuntary. This is an important result of the disease concept of alcoholism, and indeed an important reason for its promulgation. Thus special benefits are provided to alcoholism in employment, health, and civil rights law, provided they can prove that their drinking is persistent and very heavy. The effect is to reward people [for willful misconduct]. This policy is insidious precisely because it is well intended, and those who criticize it may seem to lack compassion."

From the standpoint of professional health care providers, there are also rather significant economic dimensions to the discussion. A re-definition of alcoholism as a case of willful misconduct rather than as a mental disease would, of course, relieve health insurance carriers of the obligation to reimburse expenses associated both with the burgeoning inpatient centers for alcoholism rehabilitation (some associated with psychiatric hospitals, but many free-standing) and for outpatient professional treatment.

5. Morrissey (1985, p. 96) reported that "in national surveys of the United States population . . . only 3 percent of adults report being treated for alcohol-related problems. Even among subjects who admitted experiencing interpersonal or health-related problems because of alcohol, only 19 percent of the males and 10 percent of the males had been treated."

In contrast, however, on the basis of data from the Epidemiological Catchment Area studies of the National Institute of Mental Health, Burke & Regier (1988, p. 83) reported that 12.4% of those diagnosed during the "research" interview as having alcohol abuse or dependence disorders, and 12.7% of those diagnosed as having drug abuse or dependence disorders, had sought mental health treatment within the past six months for *any* disorder, not necessarily that reflected in the focal diagnosis.

Nathan & Skinstad (1987) have reviewed in substantial detail the massive research literature on treatment for alcoholism, including demographic characteristics of treatees, treatment methods, and probable outcomes.

6. Similarly, in a study of adjudicated delinquents (70% male, 62% white) aged 16 and under judicially ordered into a "secure detention" facility in Florida, Dembo, Washburn, Wish, Schmeidler et al. (1987) found 39% to be the median drug-positive rate at admission, as assayed by EMIT methodology. These investigators further reported high congruence between self-reports of drug use and laboratory results among their subjects.

7. So long as the matter of drug use remained an issue containerized largely within criminal justice circles, little serious attention was paid by biomedical scientists to questions concerning accuracy of the various laboratory assay methods of detection, the specific biochemical laboratory procedures used to extract samples of metabolites of various controlled dangerous substances from "parent" samples, sensitivity of each method to the metabolites of various "source" substances, rates of false positives (and false negatives), and "shelf life" of samples to be analyzed. Once the matter of large scale drug testing of worker populations became an issue in the workplace, and as "cottage industries" composed of testing laboratories arose around the nation (coupled with other cottage industries which supply "alter ego" specimens to prospective examinees), however, that situation changed markedly. The journal *Seminars in Occupational Medicine*, for example, devoted its entire

December 1986 issue to substance abuse testing in the workplace (Jackson, 1986). Similarly, Dwyer (1988), of the AFL-CIO's George Meany Center for Labor Studies, has recently complained that "tests conducted on real people in the work force falsely label one of out three (32.2%) positive for drugs."

The issues here appear essentially to be a specification of the bandwidth fidelity" principle initially raised in another context by Cronbach & Glaser and recently resuscitated by Peterson (1987): *the narrower the bandwidth, the greater the fidelity of measurement.* The bandwidth fidelity argument in this context reduces to this sort of formulation: Since it is usually *not* a specific substance in the state of nature (that is, before being metabolized into a successor substance) that is discernible in post-ingestion analysis *but rather* the successor metabolite or metabolites, and since the successor substances are generally *not* uniquely related to a single source substance, it is almost certainly the case that laboratory analysis can accurately detect a specific "suspect" substance via its successor metabolite or metabolites with reasonable fidelity in a specific case *if* the immediate ingestion history of the subject is known. But it is also likely that the fidelity of detection is reduced markedly when the number of suspect substances is increased (as in broad-band laboratory assays for controlled dangerous substances of a variety of sorts, with quite different biochemical properties and metabolism routes) *and/or* when the immediate ingestion histories of large contingents of subjects are unknown — as indeed is the case in each of the laboratory assay studies reviewed here.

Without overly dwelling on the biochemistry involved, the flavor of these sets of issues can be gauged from a chapter on the forensic toxicology of cocaine by University of Utah toxicologists Finkle & McCloskey (1977, p. 169) in a National Institute on Drug Abuse Research Monograph. After noting the prospect of "thermal degradation during analysis," Finkle & McCloskey observe of EMIT technology that it "has the advantage of . . . detection of the cocaine metabolite benzoylecgonine. However, for practical purposes it is insensitive to parent cocaine."

Thus, the probability of a *false* negative *increases* when the sample to be analyzed has been extracted from the subject shortly after ingestion and before metabolizing is completed; and the issue is engaged of what other substances, whether controlled and dangerous or not, in combination with other ingested materials, are capable of producing the metabolite which EMIT technology is capable of detecting. That issue, in its turn, cannot be addressed without relatively detailed knowledge of the immediate ingestion history of the subject whose specimen is under analysis (cf. Finkle & McCloskey, 1977, p. 170).

Further, the matter is directly relevant to the burgeoning of the "designer drug" market in the U.S. If the decade between 1965 and 1975 can be characterized as the era of the narcoleptic and the hallucinogen in the U.S., that between 1975 and 1985 can be characterized as the era of the psychotomimetic, with a preference for cocaine and the amphetamines; and it seems likely that we have now entered the era of the synthetic "designer drugs." These are compounds developed in a burgeoning "cottage industry" which sets out quite consciously to avoid incorporating as an ingredient any substance which is labeled as "controlled" or "dangerous," thus producing substances that are putatively not illegal and highly resistant to detection by even the more sophisticated of the laboratory methodologies, not to say also less expensive at the point of sale and thus prospectively of wider market appeal.

The forensic implications are compelling. In a situation in which drug use may represent an aggravating factor in influencing the sanction to be imposed for a felony offense, it is surely to the prosecutor's advantage to rely on wide bandwidth testing and to minimize the prospect of alternate origins for targeted metabolites, while it is surely to defense counsel's advantage to insist on bandwidth precision in assessing the presence of unique metabolites. In the reverse situation, in which drug use represents a mitigating factor, defense counsel will prefer wide bandwidth assessment (Pallone, 1989, 1990-*a*).

8. Self-reports may be the only viable route to determining whether drug use functioned biochemically as "engine" or "lubricant" in criminal behavior, and that situation may be even further exacerbated by the availability of "designer drugs" relatively less detectable by even sophisticated laboratory assay.

To be useful to a theory of the genesis of crime, research on drug use or abuse among offenders should first establish *whether* substance use functions as *engine, lubricant,* or *motive,* and, optimally, in relation to *what* crimes.

Studies of *arrestees* may not be particularly relevant in this sphere. The acquisition of controlled dangerous substances through the proceeds of robbery or of property crime more convincingly portrays drugs as "motive" than as "engine."

Since there is no particularly strong reason to believe that those found to be drug-positive at arrest were actively "under the influence" when a crime was committed, it may be the case that they behaved criminally quite independently of what McGlothlin has called direct pharmacological influence; but there is no particular reason to believe that, either.

Only the Census study, replete with all the faults of self-report methodology and retrospective self-portrayal, but which nonetheless asked directly for a self-assessment of whether the respondent was actively "under the influence" at the time of the instant offense, responds to the question of whether controlled dangerous substances "trigger" felony crime *either* as engine or lubricant.

In view of the virtual impossibility of obtaining laboratory-analyzable data at or near the point of commission of a crime, one might well be forced to "settle" for the self-report data of convicted felons (who, after all, no longer have a strong stake in dissembling) as the most defensible approximation to a "base rate" representing whether biochemistry in fact dictated criminal behavior in an instant offense. Alternately, however, convicted felons may have a relatively strong motive for retrospective exculpation by off-loading personal guilt onto drug use.

However that may be, the relevant data suggest that something on the order of one in three felony crimes, whether of violence or against property, were at the least "lubricated" if not indeed engendered by drug use or abuse.

9. Although the American Psychiatric Association's (1984) exclusion of the effects of "voluntarily ingested" psychoactive substances, and the legislative

perpetuation of that exclusion in some states, preclude citing the toxic effects of alcohol or drugs during a period of active intoxication in support of a plea of not guilty by reason of insanity, there is as yet no impediment to citing such effects as "mitigating factors," the presence of which may not exculpate an alleged offender but may influence the severity of the sanction imposed upon conviction. In most jurisdictions, mitigating factors may include such variables as the influence of mood-altering drugs or alcohol, the prior relationship between the victim and the alleged offender, whether the victim in some way invited or colluded in his/her own victimization, etc. A litany of mitigating factors may be offset by "aggravating factors," such as the degree of demonstrable premeditation, whether the alleged criminal act was performed during the commission of another criminal act, etc.

10.   If one calculates the Yates-corrected chi square statistic to test the significance of the differences in proportions represented in the NIMH data and in the Census studies of prisoners reflected in *Figure* 12, the resultant values are each significant well beyond $p = .0001$.

4

Neurogenic Mental Disorders

Though diagnostic categories like "organic brain syndrome" have long been recognized, a state of knowledge even remotely resembling a comprehensive neuropsychiatry and neuropsychology of mental health and illness has awaited the major technological advances in the neurosciences of the relatively recent past, as highly sophisticated techniques made it possible to record brain and neurochemical activity and later to map that activity through technologically powerful imaging devices (Rosse, Owen & Morisha, 1987). A concomitant explosion of knowledge in psychopharmacology and psychoendocrinology has yielded new understandings of a panoply of interactions between brain morphology and functioning, neurochemistry, and emotional and behavioral disorder.

In the judgment of distinguished neuropsychiatrist Joseph Coyle (1988, pp. 23–24) of Johns Hopkins, the "nearly logarithmic growth in neuroscience research over the last decade" has yielded a major paradigm shift in the mental health sciences, producing in the process "new methods for diagnosing psychiatric disorders, clarifying their pathophysiology, and developing more specific and effective therapies." The net effect, according to H.M. Van Praag (1988) of the Albert Einstein College of Medicine, has been to "enable psychiatry to be a medical rather than a social science," united (or, more properly, reunited) with biology as its governing discipline.

Illustrative of current research which threatens to revolutionize traditional conceptualizations of the genesis of mental and behavioral disorder are the studies of British researchers Brown, Colter, Corsellis, Crow et al. (1986), who found evidence at autopsy of structural brain changes particularly involving the temporal lobe among schizophrenic patients, and Harvard neuropsychiatrists Cohen, Buonanno, Keck, Finklestein & Benes (1988), who identified through computerized tomography (CT) scans and magnetic resonance imaging (MRI) techniques consistent neuroanatomical anomalies in depressive and schizophrenic patients, even though "standard" neurological exam- inations had failed to detect these abnormalities in 63% of the cases. Similarly, at the Neurosciences Laboratory of the National Institute of Mental Health, Luxenberg, Swedo, Flament, Friedland, Rapoport & Rapoport (1988) identified through CT scans consistent neuroana- tomical abnormality in patients diagnosed as obsessive-compulsive.

The evidence on the neurogenesis of schizophrenia, the most insidi- ous of the mental disorders, is now quite impressive.[1] In a major review of that evidence, University of Maryland neuropsychiatrists Heinrichs & Buchanan (1988, pp. 16–17) conclude:

> In spite of some methodological limitations, the evidence for a higher rate of neurological abnormalities in schizophrenia is consistent and compelling. These signs are not random but are concentrated in the functional domains of sensory integration, coordination, and sequen- tial motor acts. There is some suggestion that these functional systems are impaired at the level of subcortical structures such as the limbic system. Furthermore, there are indications that neurological signs are more prominent among those with thought disorder and cogni- tive impairments, as well as those with chronic forms of the illness. In addition, there is significant reason to believe that neurological abnormalities characterize a portion of the relatives of schizophrenic patients and *predate* the onset of the schizophrenic illness.

While interviews by non-specialists or administration of paper-and- pencil instruments might suffice in cataloging the relative incidence of "psychological" disorders, assessment of neuropsychiatric, psy- chopharmacological, and psychoendocrinological disorders requires detailed laboratory examination, often utilizing expensive medical instrumentation for imaging studies. It is not surprising, therefore, that no contemporary census has been attempted of the overall prevalence of such disorders in the general population. Indeed, among the several early mental health surveys reviewed in Chapter 2, Pasamanick's (1962) study alone attended to organic mental disorder as a distinct cate- gory, with a prevalence rate in the general population of 0.14%. Since Pasamanick's subjects underwent "thorough clinical and laboratory evaluations at the Johns Hopkins Hospital," his data emanated from methods of assessment that were scientifically sound for their time. Since the succeeding years have produced significantly more advanced methods of assessment, however, it is virtually certain that that ratio represents an underestimate by current scientific standards. If the "false negative" ratio embedded in the study by Cohen, Buonanno, Keck,

Finklestein & Benes (1988) is applied to Pasamanick's prevalence data, it is likely that the underestimate is minimally on the order of 270%; but even application of that ratio as a corrective factor to Pasamanick's data suggests an incidence in the general population no higher than 0.4%.

Because disordered brain and neurochemical processes often eventuate in violent behavior, however, and because subjects with a history of violence are to be found in great profusion in prison populations, many studies of the relationship between neurological disorder and violence have been conducted within correctional settings, with offenders convicted of violent crimes as subjects. These studies have contributed directly to the emerging picture of the neurogenesis of violence, but have not in the main attempted to assay the overall prevalence of neurogenic mental disorder in the correctional population.

Organic Disorders and Violent Behavior

Though there is no imputation that organicity represents an exclusive "cause," a wide panoply of organic disorders has been empirically determined to be related to violent behavior, whether formally criminal or not. Neuropsychiatrist Kenneth Tardiff (1988, p. 1042) of the Medical College at Cornell has summarized the accumulated evidence:

> A number of organic disorders are associated with violent behavior, including substance abuse, central nervous system disorders, systemic disorders, and seizure disorders. Central nervous system disorders which have been associated with violent behavior include traumatic brain injuries, including birth injury as well as trauma as an adult acutely and in the post-concussion syndrome; intracranial infections; cerebrovascular disorders; Alzheimer's disease [a degenerative brain disorder primarily affecting the cerebral cortex]; Wilson's disease [a disorder of liver functioning]; multiple sclerosis. Systemic disorders affecting the central nervous system include metabolic disorders such as hypoglycemia, vitamin deficiencies, electrolyte imbalances, hypoxia [a pulmonary disorder], uremia, Cushing's anemia, systemic infections, systemic lupus erythematosus, porphyria, and industrial poisons such as lead.

In a less expansive catalog, British neuropsychologist Rodger [sic] Llewellyn Wood (1987, pp. 21–22) attributes aggressiveness to injury to the frontal lobes of the brain, thought to be the seat of memory, concentration, abstraction, and judgment. Aggressive episodes are said to result from "some paroxysmal electrical event," so that "Once started, the patient seems to have little or no control over the course of behaviour." Moreover, "Diminished insight is an almost inevitable consequence of severe frontal lobe injury" (p. 25).

George Whatmore and Daniel Kohli (1974), specialists in internal medicine, trace the sources of uncontrollable rage (or what they call "dyslimbic anger") to anomalies in neuromuscular pathways, such that "repetitive excitatory effects" are produced in the limbic portion of the central nervous system, with the result that repetitive excitatory signals in the limbic system magnify "anger-activating signals to produce exaggerated anger" (p. 109).

Joseph (1990, pp. 96–103) similarly attributes aggressivity to dysfunctions in limbic system structures, particularly the hypothalamus and the amygdala, citing experimental evidence on both animal and human subjects of the effects of electrical stimulation on these structures in producing behavior very similar to that described by Felson & Steadman (1982) in their social psychological analysis of "situational variables" in criminal violence.[2]

Brain Function Anomalies

In the source described as the "most widely used medical text in the world," Berkow & Fletcher (1987, p. 1366) define epilepsy as "A recurrent paroxysmal disorder of cerebral function characterized by sudden, brief attacks of altered consciousness, motor activity, sensory phenomena, or inappropriate behavior," and go on to note that, beyond the *grand mal* seizures commonly seen and readily identifiable even to medically untrained observers, "any recurrent seizure pattern may be termed epilepsy." They trace the etiology to sources as diverse as microscopic scars on brain tissue resultant from birth trauma or head injury, central nervous system infection, metabolic dysfunctions (including hypoglycemia), ingestion of toxins (including alcohol and hypnotic or tranquilizing drugs), brain lesions and defects, and cerebral edema of the sort common in concussion. Though on the order of some 85% of all cases can be diagnosed through electroencephalographic (EEG), computerized tomography, or magnetic resonance imaging techniques, in the remaining cases "the diagnosis of epilepsy as opposed to a behavioral [i.e., functional psychological] disorder may have to be made on clinical grounds" (*Ibid.*, pp. 1369–1370). Cases in the latter category, which may be fully confirmed only at autopsy, have come to be called conditions of "subclinical severity."

Current leading scientific opinion in neuropsychiatry relates head trauma, often unreported and untreated, to a variety of consequent mental disorders, including "confusion, intellectual changes, affective lability, or psychosis . . . substance abuse, impulse disorders, and characterological disorders, such as antisocial, borderline, and narcissistic personality disorders," although and very significantly, "the cognitive functions of the patient are preserved" (Silver, Yudofsky & Hales, 1987, p. 180).

Similarly, head trauma resultant in even subclinical epilepsy or epileptiform disorder, is said to perpetuate as organic personality syndrome, further differentiated into "pseudo-psychopathic (characterized by emotional lability, impulsivity, socially inappropriate behavior, and hostility) and pseudo-depressive (characterized by apathy, indifference, and social disconnectedness)," with both syndromes "marked by indifference for the consequences of behavior and an inability to perceive appropriately the effects of such behavior on others" (Stoudemire, 1987, pp. 134–135).

The latter characteristics (i.e., indifference to the consequences of behavior, disregard of the social impact of one's own behavior), indeed, are virtually the defining traits embedded in classic conceptions of psychopathy (Hare, 1985; Heilbrun & Heilbrun, 1985; Meloy, 1988).

In a study that provided further confirmation of Stoudemire's (1987) view that closed head injury perpetuates as organic personality disorder either of the "pseudo-depressive" or "pseudo-psychopathic" variety, Fletcher, Ewing-Cobbs, Miner, Levin & Eisenberg (1990) followed for a year a group of children aged between 3 and 15 who had sustained closed head injuries and had been treated in the children's pediatric neurosurgery service at the University of Texas' Houston medical campus. Data collected by means of structured checklists completed by parents (the Vineland Adaptive Behavior Scales, the Child Behavior Checklist) indicated that negative behavioral effects associated with the head injuries persisted throughout the follow-up period; those effects ranged from "quiet withdrawal to hyperactive, aggressive behavior," (p. 97).

Moreover, persons who have suffered past head trauma frequently fail to link such trauma to current disorders (Silver, Yudoksky & Hales, 1987, p. 180):

> Prototypic examples of brain damage in which the patient, while providing a [psychiatric] history may fail to associate [current symptoms] with the traumatic event include the alcoholic who is amnestic for a fall that occurred while inebriated; the 10-year-old boy whose head was hit while falling from his bicycle, but who fails to inform

his parents; or the wife who was beaten by her husband, but who is either fearful or ashamed to report the injury to her family physician. Such trauma may be associated with confusion, intellectual changes, affective lability, or psychosis; and the patient may first present [these latter symptoms] to the psychiatrist for evaluation and treatment.

Further, victims of head trauma, particularly that which has been undetected, diagnosed imprecisely, or minimized, are "prone to the taking of risks," so that a vicious circle develops, since risk-takers are attracted to activities that entail a high probability for further head trauma (*Ibid.*, pp. 180–181). Hence, victims of head trauma are at risk for risk-taking behavior which further increases the probability of future, additional head trauma, and which, in its turn, increases the likelihood of future risk-taking behavior *ad infinitum*.

That circle begins to sound very much like the "tinder box" circumstances that surround 60% of the episodes of criminal homicide in this country, reviewed in Chapter 3.

Studies among Offenders

An array of investigations has studied the incidence of brain and brain-bioelectrical anomalies among samples of incarcerated criminal offenders,[3] usually by means of technologically sophisticated medical instruments but sometimes by means of complex neuropsychological test batteries that have been concurrently well validated against such "hands on" technology (Franzen & Lovell, 1987). Particularly in those cases in which data have been gathered through advanced imaging techniques, the samples in these studies tend to be rather small, so that the resultant conclusions can be generalized only with great caution. Nonetheless:

- The incidence of epilepsy among prisoners incarcerated for criminal behavior of all sorts significantly exceeds that of control subjects matched for age (Wettstein, 1987, p. 458). In a study of all new adult male admissions to the Illinois state prisons utilizing comprehensive neurological examinations, including EEG readings, Whitman, Coleman, Patmon, Desai, Cohen & King (1984) found the rate of epilepsy among prisoners to be four times higher than the incidence in a comparably aged group of non-prisoners and further opined on the basis of case history data that head trauma likely accounted for epilepsy in 45% of the cases detected.
- The incidence of undetected and untreated closed head trauma, likely indicative of brain dysfunction of at least a subclinical level of severity, is substantially higher among members of lower socioeconomic status

groups and among blacks, two groups among whom commission of crimes of violence also shows a higher incidence (Bell, 1986).

- Howard (1984) took electroencephalograph readings of consecutive admissions to a prison hospital in Britain, with the finding that atypical brain activity was recorded in 60% of the cases. Howard further observed that particular anomalies in brain functioning were prevalent in subjects who had committed crimes of violence against strangers rather than against friends or acquaintances. His finding is clinically corroborated in a study by Martinius (1983) of criminal homicide.

- Blackburn (1975, 1979) found electroencephalographic (EEG) evidence of abnormally high cortical arousal among prisoners diagnosed as "primary psychopaths." These subjects also scored significantly higher than controls on psychometric measures of "sensation seeking" and susceptibility to boredom, so that Blackburn's results support at a basic physiological level Hare's (1970) view that hyperarousability is a distinguishing characteristic of psychopaths.

- Similarly, Gorenstein (1982) found evidence among subjects classified as psychopaths on behavioral and psychometric criteria of dysfunction in the frontal lobe of the brain, thought to be associated with such psychological functions as foresight, planning, and the regulation of impulses.[4]

- Parallel findings were reported by Krakowski, Convit, Jaeger & Lin (1989) in studies of schizophrenics with a history of criminal violence, verified by EEG readings, leading these investigators to conclude that "violence as well as neurological and neuropsychological deficits characterize a more severe form of schizophrenia."

- Raine & Venables (1988) similarly reported anomalies in parietal lobe functioning as measured by EEG among inmates diagnosed as psychopathic.

- In a rare instance in which evidence of brain dysfunction was available on a large birth cohort, Petersen, Matousek, Mednick et al. (1982) reported that "previous EEG abnormalities" detected in childhood or early adolescence were associated with later criminal behavior. Similarly, Virkkunen, Nuutila & Huusko (1976) followed a sample of brain-injured World War II veterans for nearly 30 years, concluding that the incidence of later criminality was associated with injury to the frontotemporal region; importantly, they found that "the criminal acts very often happened only after several decades following the head injury."

- In a study that compared EEG readings, CT scans of the brain, and results of the Luria-Nebraska Neuropsychological test battery, Langevin, Ben-Aron, Wortzman & Dickey (1987), found "a consistent trend toward more neuropathology" in violent and assaultive offenders than in offenders who were guilty of property crimes; but, perhaps in a manner that explains weak statistical associations between inventoried personality traits and criminal violence, these differences in neuropathology were *not* matched by differences in psychometric profiles on the Minnesota Multiphasic Personality Inventory.[5]

- Yeudall & Fromm-Auch (1979) found evidence of neuropathology through administration of a comprehensive neuropsychological battery in 94% of the homicide offenders, 96% of the sex offenders, 89% of the assaulters, and 86% of the juvenile offenders they examined, with these findings confirmed by subsequent EEG readings. Congruent findings were reported by Spellacy (1978), who also reported that neuropsychological assessment discriminated between violent and non-violent prisoners more effectively than did results of the MMPI. Similarly, though they employed only clinical neuropsychological test measures rather than medical neurological assessment devices, Bryant, Scott, Tori & Golden (1984) found consistent associations between neuropsychological deficit and a history of violent criminal behavior. In a retrospective that eventuated in a new conceptualization of persistent criminal behavior as triggered by interaction between biological, social, and psychological contributors, Yeudall, Fedora & Fromm (1987) reviewed data on the incidence of head injury among alcoholic psychopaths (77%), homicide offenders (75%), rapists (21 %), and offenders who had committed physical assault (25%).
- In an extensive investigation that involved both administration of a comprehensive neuropsychological test battery, measures of penile tumescence in response to erotic stimuli of varying character (male/female, adult/child), and CT scans of the brain, Hucker, Langevin, Wortzman & Bain (1986) found a high incidence of neuropathology, particularly involving the left temporoparietal region of the brain, among subjects whose criminal histories classified them as focused pedophiles.
- Similarly, at the Kessler Institute for Rehabilitation Medicine, Galski, Thornton & Shumsky (1990) found evidence of significant neuropsychological dysfunction in 77% of the incarcerated criminal sexual psychopaths they examined on the Luria Nebraska Neuropsychological battery, discovering as well so strong an association between neuropsychological impairment and the degree of violence associated with the most recent sex offense that they were led to conclude that "violent sexual offenses seem to be linked with more severe neuropsychological dysfunction, specifically associated with left hemisphere functioning," thought to control (at least among those who are right handed) such functions as sequential and analytic processing of ideas and concepts (Taylor, Sierles & Abrams, 1987, pp. 4–5).

Neurochemical Anomalies

More fundamentally, the role of basic neuropharmacology and neuroendocrinology in violent behavior, whether such behavior be adjudicated as formally criminal or not, is only now beginning to be understood. A wide range of psychopharmacological and psychoendocrinologic research on offender groups has been reported and is underway, much of it in Scandinavian countries, and, because of the extensive laboratory protocols necessarily involved (e.g., many studies of the metabolism of neural transmitting enzymes require samples of spinal fluid, available only through surgical lumbar puncture), typically limited to small groups of subjects. Scattered studies yield fragmentary evidence that coalesces to produce a picture that may be indicative but is not yet definitive. Nonetheless, a number of studies point toward a prospective relationship between anomalies in neurochemistry and aggressive behavior:

- In studies of violent offenders across types of crime, Matti Virkkunnen (1982-*a*, *b*, 1983-*a*, 1984, 1985, 1986, 1987, 1989) and his colleagues at the University of Helsinki have found evidence for the *abnormal metabolism of glucose*, an excess of which can produce "manic" states, especially among those diagnosed with antisocial personality disorder. Though their subjects had no particular history of criminal behavior, Gur, Resnick, Gur, Alavi et al. (1987) also found anomalies in the metabolism of cerebral glucose, especially in the left hemisphere of the brain, among schizophrenic patients (but not among non-schizophrenic controls) studied at the University of Pennsylvania using positron emission tomography (PET).
- Several investigators (Bradford & McLean, 1984; Dabbs, Frady, Carr & Besch, 1987; Rada & Kellner, 1976; Rada, Kellner, Stivastava & Peake, 1983; Virkkunen, 1985) have reported *abnormally high concentrations of testosterone among inmates with a history of violent crime*, whether these were sexually focused or not. Pertinently to correctional treatment or control considerations, testosterone levels are amenable to biochemical manipulation through hormone-suppressing agents.
- Boulton, Davis, Yu et al. (1983), Lidberg (1985), and Virkkunen, Nuutila, Goodwin & Linnoila (1987) have found evidence of the *abnormal metabolism of monoamine oxidase*, an important neural transmitter that regulates mood, the inhibition of which indeed constitutes the biochemical basis for many antidepressant psychotropic medications (Schatzberg & Cole, 1986, pp. 46–54), leading to the tentative conclusion of *an enduring relationship between impaired impulse control and naturally occurring anomalies in the body's regulation of neural transmission.*
- At Eastern Pennsylvania Psychiatric Institute, Coccaro, Siever, Klar & Maurer (1989) reported abnormal metabolism of serotonin, a powerful neurotransmitter directly related to the psychobiology of depression, among subjects with a history of impulsive aggression who had been independently diagnosed as psychopathic. Similar results were reported by Virkkunen & Narvanen (1987) in a more complex study

that also traced the interactive effects between insulin, tryptophan, and serotonin.

- At a primitive molecular level, Virkkunen, Horrobin, Jenkins & Manku (1987), through analysis of cerebrospinal fluid, found anomalies in the production of prostacyclin, an ubiquitous metabolite of unsaturated fatty acids that in turn directly affects the metabolism of the powerful neurotransmitter norepinephrine and itself directly influences the perception of pain, among violent offenders diagnosed with antisocial personality disorder.

In a multidimensional study that suggests the interaction of extrinsic forces and intrinsic neurochemical factors in the generation of violent behavior that extended Virkkunen's (1979) earlier work on the effects of alcohol on violence in subjects who had been diagnosed with antisocial personality disorder, Virkkunen, Nuutila, Goodwin & Linnoila (1987) observed a high rate of alcoholism among violent offenders in whom they had also observed anomalies in regulation of neural transmitters and opined that, because ingestion of alcohol represents a temporary corrective to abnormal metabolism of monoamine oxidase, "*alcohol abuse* in these individuals . . . *may represent an effort to self-medicate,*" even though "alcohol only makes the situation worse by further impairing impulse control." In other studies, Virkkunen and his colleagues have observed a relationship between habitual violence and abnormal metabolism of cholesterol (1983) and abnormal metabolism of glucose (1987) *under the influence of* alcohol. Nonetheless, it will patently be the case that, whether at the scene of a crime or in later studies which rely on social history variables, violent behavior will be attributed to alcohol ingestion; the issue of why it seems to a particular abuser of alcohol that he or she "feels better" when drinking (i.e., the issue of whether alcohol use or abuse is itself an effort to self-medicate and thus *secondary* to a naturally occurring neuro-anomaly) will scarcely be raised.

Cause, Effect, or Concomitant?

Though the evidence of a statistical association (technically, no more than a correlative association) between bioelectrical or neurochemical anomalies and violent criminal behavior is relatively strong, the state of the evidence does not yet permit determination of precedent and antecedent (much less, of "cause and effect") relationships. Such determination would require, as Heinrichs & Buchanan (1987) observed in regard to the evidence on the neurogenesis of schizophrenia, clear indication that neurophysiological dysfunction "predates" criminal violence.

As Robert Wettstein (1988, p. 1066), a leading forensic psychiatrist at the University of Pittsburgh, has put the matter in respect of the prospective relationships between epilepsy and criminal violence:

> [S]everal relationships between antisocial conduct and epilepsy can be inferred: a) antisocial act caused by a seizure; b) cerebral malfunction causing both epilepsy and antisocial behavior; c) antisocial behavior resulting in low self-esteem and social rejection suffered by patients with epilepsy; d) antisocial behavior symptomatic of a mental disorder as a result of epilepsy; e) psychosocial environmental deprivations causing both epilepsy and antisocial behavior; and f) antisocial behavior which produces accidental brain trauma.

The directionality of the relationship is complicated by the relative insensitivity of even highly sophisticated measuring devices to the time of onset of brain dysfunction, except perhaps in cases of very recent head trauma, typically independently verifiable from physical evidence of concussion. Though most knowledgeable commentators would regard neurochemical anomalies as constitutional or congenital rather than acquired through accident or injury, the regulation of neurotransmitting fluids may be affected by brain dysfunctions consequent to injury sustained during violent behavior; thus, the issue of directionality may apply as well to anomalies in neurochemical processing.

There is also the issue of the interaction between brain dysfunction, substance abuse, and violence, as Virkkunen, Nuutila, Goodwin & Linnoila (1987) have suggested. Hence, people who over-imbibe alcohol (or use psychotomimetic drugs) tend to find themselves in violence-prone situations; people in violence-prone situations are susceptible to head injury, whether from fights with others also intoxicated or from the business end of a police officer's night stick; alternately, simple intoxication may lead to falls that engender head injury or compound pre-existing dysfunctions.

A Tinder Box Writ Large?

Sociological interpretations of criminal violence would tend to support an interactive hypothesis. After investigating the confluence of suicide, homicide, and violent crime in the several regions of the nation, Gastil (1971) proposed that a "subculture of violence," liberally lubricated by alcohol use or abuse, pervaded the American South. Doerner (1975), Bailey (1976), and Humphrey & Kupferer (1977) provided confirmatory evidence.

In more discerning analyses of nearly 500 "standard metropolitan statistical areas" in the U.S., Messner (1982, 1983, 1985) concluded that the propensity for violent death appears to pervade the population of that region, regardless of race or economic deprivation. Surely, that is a picture of "tinder box" circumstances writ large; but that subculture begins to sound very much as if it were peopled by the "risk takers" described by Silver, Yudofsky & Hales (1987), whose propensities for violence were said to inhere in brain dysfunction.[6]

Intergenerational Transmission of Neurogenic Violence

Yet, unless it be demonstrated that one uniform child care practice in such a subculture of violence requires dropping infants on their heads from great heights or otherwise engendering head injury, it seems less likely that brain disorder uniformly constitutes a condition *precedent* to violent behavior, even in a subculture prone to violence, than that brain disorder constitutes a condition *consequent* to a lifestyle rich in violent behavior, replete with ample social supports.

Nonetheless, one would expect that child rearing practices in such a subculture would favor (or at least condone) physical punishment as a means of behavior control. Especially in light of Bell's (1986) findings on the incidence of head trauma in relation to social class, the prospect that such class-linked child rearing practices may yield a higher incidence of "accidental" head injury (and thus also of consequent neuropsychological dysfunction) cannot be dismissed out of hand.

Some support for such an interpretation emerges from studies by Tarter, Hegedus, Winsten & Alterman (1984) on neuropsychological impairment among juvenile delinquents who had themselves been the victims of parental physical abuse; by Wolfe, Fairbank, Kelly & Bradlyn (1983) on autonomic arousal levels in relation to videotaped depictions of even non-stressful interactions between parents and children on the part of physically abusive mothers; and by Rohrbeck & Twentyman (1986) on neuropsychological deficits among abusive mothers.

To the extent to which Cloninger, Reich & Guze (1975) were correct in proposing that psychopathy is intergenerationally transmitted and further compounded by a process they call "associative mating" (whereby individuals choose spouses not very different from themselves), it may be that harsh child rearing practices in a subculture that condones violence constitutes an important intervening biopsychosocial variable.

However engaging at the conceptual level, the question of directionality is significant primarily to a theory of criminogenesis. At the practical level of correctional management, the mere *fact* that propensities for violent behavior co-exist with brain dysfunctions is the salient issue, whatever the direction of the relationship.

The Question of Culpability Revisited

The scientific picture on the neurogenesis (as distinct from the biogenesis, at least in the sense of inherited constitutional predispositions, as Herrnstein [1990] appears to understand the term) of violence is currently richly suggestive but not yet definitive. Given what is currently either known or hypothesized about brain and neurochemical anomalies thought to "control" impulsivity and aggression, and in light of at least fragmentary evidence about the incidence of anomalies in brain and neurochemical functioning among violent offenders, it may well be the case that future research will demonstrate conclusively that criminally aggressive behavior is "triggered" by very primitive neurophysiological or neurochemical processes over which the individual can be expected to exert little *volitional* control.

Some rather silly academic debates about antecedent and consequent conditions — concerning whether, for example, such personality traits as are measurable through psychometric or clinical instruments result from disordered neuropsychological processes or whether such traits (presumably acquired as the remnants of disordered developmental or learning processes) dictate disordered neuropsychological processes — might then be expected. But the more salient debates will concern the implications of revolutionized understandings of the genesis of violent behavior that is formally criminal for societal and legislative notions of culpability, as Wilson & Herrnstein (1985, pp. 504–505) have somewhat satirically foreseen:

> If society should not punish acts that science has shown to have been caused by antecedent conditions, then every advance in knowledge about why people behave as they do may shrink the scope of criminal law. If, for example, it is shown that [violent] offenders suffer from abnormal hormones combined with certain atypical relations with their parents, then, by the existing standards of responsibility, why should their attorneys not demand acquittal on grounds of bad hormones combined with a particular family history?

Moreover, the matter of directionality may not be pertinent in fixing culpability for a particular offense, unless it be the case that the putatively "triggering" brain or neurochemical anomaly can be demonstrated to have arisen *consequent* to that offense. Consider a situation, for example, in which earlier, documented episodes of criminal violence have yielded neuropsychological anomalies of such character that the emission of violent behavior is virtually beyond the control of the individual, and in which there is also documented evidence that the individual in question was free of such anomalies prior to those earlier episodes. In an *instant* case of criminal violence *subsequent* to the onset of such anomalies, what degree of culpability should attach to that individual? In that situation, whether the earlier episodes of violent behavior that "caused" those anomalies themselves constituted "willful misconduct" may be quite irrelevant.

Though a formal diagnosis of "organic psychosis" as the perpetuation of brain or neurochemical disorder would seem to fit within legislatively established criteria for non-culpability, most current formulations of the criteria for culpability and exculpation as reflected in the M'Naghten Standard and its variants are not readily applicable to cases in which criminal behavior is triggered by brain or neurochemical dysfunction.

Quite clearly, advances in knowledge about the neurogenesis of violence will inevitably "shrink the scope of criminal law" — indeed, as effectively as the scope of the law underwent shrinkage a century and a half ago when then-current scientific knowledge led to the initial formulation of the M'Naghten Standard. In particular, the exclusion of psychopathic deviation (i.e., that "the terms 'mental disease or defect' do not include an abnormality manifested only by repeated antisocial conduct") in the American Law Institute's formulation (reviewed in Chapter 3) needs substantial discerning reconsideration in the light of evidence that links, even correlatively, criminal violence with neurophysiological and neurochemical dysfunction.

Correctional Management of Neurogenic Violence

If such reconsideration maintains the current narrow grounds for exculpation, responsibility for the management of neurogenically violent offenders will remain within the province of correctional institutions. If such reconsideration results in a broadening of the grounds for exculpation, responsibility for the management of offenders whose criminal violence has been triggered neurogenically will likely be transferred from the province of correctional institutions to that of the mental hospitals. Hence, whatever the result of the inevitable conceptual debates as the evidence for the neurogenesis of criminal violence accumulates, at the practical level the matter of methods of control remains at issue.

Neither set of institutions seems presently well prepared to accommodate the major paradigm shift that has yielded "new methods for diagnosing psychiatric disorders, clarifying their pathophysiology, and developing more specific and effective therapies," of which Coyle (1988) has spoken. If neurogenic criminally violent behavior is to be effectively managed, it seems clear that the methods of management must address such behavior at its molar roots, utilizing precisely those "specific and effective" methods that have emerged from the explosion in neuroscientific knowledge.

Neurosurgery in Neurogenic Aggression

As an illustration, consider a case of "quite savage acts of aggression" managed neither in a correctional facility nor a psychiatric hospital but rather at the Kemsley Unit of St. Andrew's Hospital, Northampton, England, a medical installation for the rehabilitation of head trauma. The methods employed correspond neither to those standard in correctional facilities (i.e., externally applied behavior control) nor to those standard in mental hospitals (i.e., psychotropic medication combined with supportive psychotherapy). Instead, following the *failure* of a regimen consisting of pharmacotherapy and behavior therapy, effective management required application of advanced neurosurgery, as described by Wood (1987, p. 72):

> [An] aggressive behavior pattern . . . occurred in a 19-year-old patient who had sustained a severe head injury 28 months earlier. He had no serious physical sequelae . . . From admission, the patient was known to have an abnormal EEG, suggesting that an electrical anomaly was responsible for his unprovoked, volatile outbursts which included quite savage acts of aggression . . . This [condition] was treated from admission by a combination of carbamazepine [a medication intended for the relief of epileptic seizures, usually marketed under the trade name Tegretol] and behaviour management. There was, however, only a temporary reduction in aggressive behaviour and, instead of continuing to improve, his behaviour deteriorated. It was then noticed that the patient had intermittent nasal discharge of cerebrospinal fluid (CSF). Neurological investigations showed that this intermittent CSF discharge was due to increases in intra-cranial pressure, forcing CSF through a tear in the dura [the fibrous membrane covering the brain and spinal cord]. The build-up of pressure within the skull probably

precipitated an electrical discharge in the limbic system, profoundly affecting behaviour. The patient was transferred back to a neurosurgical unit long enough for a ventriculo-peritoneal shunt to be inserted. The frequency of aggression before and after the shunt operation to reduce intra-cranial pressure [was] very different . . . confirming that neurological, not psychological, factors were responsible for the aggressive behavior.

Because the surgery performed in this case remediated a medically-verified neurological impairment (itself the result of accidental injury), the regimen followed differs fundamentally from the "serious and indiscriminate destruction of brain tissue [that] would render almost any offender so incapacitated as to be unable to think or act with sufficient efficiency to engage in . . . criminal behavior" properly vilified by Halleck (1987, p. 175) as ethically unacceptable in the treatment of offenders, or anyone else.

Cognitive Rehabilitation and Impulse Control

Though less dramatically, a variety of techniques for *cognitive rehabilitation,* often based on computerization and programmed learning, have been developed by neuropsychologists in treatment facilities for patients with head injury (or, less often, those suffering the effects of prolonged biochemical insult to the brain through the use of alcohol or virulently psychotomimetic substances) in medical installations devoted to brain injury rehabilitation (Franzen & Sullivan, 1987; Yohman, Schaeffer & Parsons, 1988). Not to be confused with cognitive-behavior therapy, cognitive rehabilitation techniques constitute a sophisticated method of "teaching" patients to compensate for cognitive functions which have been damaged as a consequence of injury to brain tissues "using the learning theory concepts of componential learning, approximation, and reinforcement for success" (Franzen & Sullivan, 1987, p. 443).

Cognitive rehabilitation regimens have been successful in addressing deficits in memory and problem-solving capacity but are also employable to retrain patients with impairments in impulse control, by "teaching" patients to increase their attention span, inhibit urges to behave, foresee consequences, and consider alternatives. In the aggregate, these techniques derive from a knowledge base in clinical neuropsychology rooted in the psychology of learning rather from the armamentarium of psychotherapy.

The following case, treated at the Robert Wood Johnson Life-style Institute in New Jersey, an installation specializing in rehabilitation medicine, illustrates the application of these techniques to problems in impulse control (Cicerone & Wood, 1987, pp. 111–112):

> The client is a 20 year old right-handed man who had sustained a closed head injury in a motor vehicle accident four years earlier. Computed tomography performed shortly after his hospital admission showed multiple contusions, right cerebral edema with right to left midline shift, and a right frontal intracerebral hematoma . . . There was continued improvement over the next three months . . . More recently, the family became concerned over his marked impulsivity and interpersonal difficulties. He frequently interrupted conversations with other family members and friends, his own speech became expansive and circumstantial, and it often appeared as if "he doesn't think before he does something." Initial neuropsychological evaluation was conducted four years after his injury . . . Neuropsychological evaluations were most notable for marked impaired of planning ability and difficulty evaluating results of his own actions [and] disturbances of "higher executive functions" (e.g., initiation, planning, and self-regulation) . . . Treatment was based on a modified self-instructional procedure which required him to verbalize a plan before and during execution of the training task and then to gradually fade overt verbalization. The training task was a modified version of the "Tower of London," which requires the subject to move three different color beads onto three different sized pegs from a specified starting position in a restricted number of moves. . . The self-instructional training was conducted in three stages. Throughout the course of training, the client received general instructions about various aspect of planning and problem solving, e.g., problem formulation, goal definition, subgoal identification, consideration of alternatives, and self-evaluation of results . . . A major concern of the cognitive training was generalization of treatment effects to everyday behavior . . . there was an implicit demand for self-monitoring built into the training procedure. Replication of real-life examples during treatment allowed the client to compare his behavior in those situations with the solution he arrived at using the treatment strategy. He could also evaluate any discrepancy between his actual and planned solutions.

A variety of psychometric measures demonstrated not only significant improvement in the *in vitro* tasks at hand but generalization of effect to a wide array of "real life" situations, with a "systematic reduction and eventual cessation in target behaviors" during the course of training and during a follow-up period.

Non-Therapeutic Use of Mood-Altering Substances

On the basis of their own research and that of others on the neu-rochemistry of criminal violence, Virkkunen, Nuutila, Good-win & Linnoila (1987, pp. 245–246) seem to hold that even the present state of knowledge yields important implications for the pharmacological management of violent offenders:

> [Deficiencies in a metabolite of monoamine oxidase are] associated with aggression dyscontrol by being conducive of a heightened aggressive drive . . . more specifically with a deficiency of impulse control and because of this with dyscontrol of intrapersonal and interpersonal aggression . . . Aggressivity and impulse control problems are very closely related, especially in violent offenders . . . In controlled clinical studies, both tryptophan and lithium carbonate have been found to be effective in reducing violent acts by habitually impulsive and violent offenders, and by adolescents with undersocialized aggressive conduct disorders characterized by severe aggressiveness and explosive impulsivity . . . Thus, it seems that lithium carbonate may rather specifically ameliorate impulse control problems.

The implications might seem to flow in the direction of the administration of psychotropic medication in those settings charged with the management of neurogenically violent offenders. But the right of patients (even involuntarily committed patients) to refuse medication for the treatment of mental illness, deriving from "the basic assumption in our society that all persons have the right to control intrusions on their bodies" (Appelbaum, 1988, p. 413), has now been firmly established (Brooks, 1986; Rodenhauser, 1984) and in Lar*ge v. Superior Court* (714 P.2D 399, Arizona, 1986) and *People v. Delgado* (A042371, First Appellate District, California, 1989), state courts had specifically extended that right to prisoners as well. Moreover, it is a reasonable speculation that some portion of neurogenically violent offenders would regard their disorders as ego-syntonic and thus perceive themselves as scarcely in need of pharmacotherapeutic treatment for a condition they do *not* perceive as an abnormality.[7]

However, in a decision announced on February 27, 1990 (*Washington v. Harper*, 88–599), the scope of which is really quite limited but would seem to include neurogenically violent offenders, the U.S. Supreme Court opened a "window" on the matter of *involuntary* administration of psychotropic medication to prisoners. The specific case concerned the acceptability under the Constitution of the procedures used in the

State of Washington to determine whether psychoactive medication should be administered to an inmate against his or her will. Those procedures require the decision of a review board composed of a prison psychiatrist, a prison psychologist, and a correctional administrator to overrule the inmate's declination; the inmate has the right to be represented by an advisor but not by an attorney.[8] The key phrases in the Supreme Court's decision hold that the state is constitutionally permitted (with emphases added) "to treat a prison inmate who has a serious mental illness with antipsychotic drugs against his will, *if the inmate is dangerous to himself or others.*"

Clearly, it is the "clear and imminent danger" test[9] that has been applied by the Court in its reasoning, so that the scope of the decision appears limited to those situations in which an inmate presents an imminent threat of violence *within* the correctional setting.

That is a situation at some considerable conceptual and operational distance from the involuntary administration of medication to treat a disorder *on account of which* an inmate has become an inmate but which cannot reasonably be linked to the prospect of suicide or assault while in custody — as, for example, in the administration of hormone-suppressing pharmacologic agents to focused pedophiles confined judicially for treatment, but in an institution for adults, a class of victim toward whom such offenders have shown no prior violent disposition.

Even though the scope of *Washington v. Harper* would seem to preclude such aggressive pharmacotherapy as, for example, chemical castration by means of hormone-suppressing pharmacological agents in the *rehabilitative* treatment of sex offenders (Pallone, 1990-*b*, pp. 85–86), the window has been opened for future litigation — perhaps, indeed, brought by sex offenders as *plaintiffs* who would prefer chemical castration (followed by release) to continued confinement for treatment that is non-pharmacotherapeutic.

There is every reason to believe, however, that neurogenically violent offenders in custody (and, more particularly, those for whom there is corroborative evidence, as from the MMPI, that mania and impulsivity are characteristic patterns of behavior) would fall precisely within the scope of *Harper.* Even so, there may be other ways to deliver the mood-altering substances cited by Virkkunen, Nuutila, Goodwin & Linnoila which do *not* require the administration of psychotropic medication.

Tryptophan on the Menu?

Tryptophan is an amino acid which directly affects the metabolism of brain serotonin, a powerful neurotransmitter and neural regulator; one current hypothesis on the genesis of disorders of affect attributes their source to functional deficiencies in the metabolism of a tryptophan by-product (Martin, Owen & Morisha, 1987, pp. 69–71; Cowen, 1988). The substance is also implicated in the body's production of dietary niacin; niacin deficiency (pellagra) produces such behavioral sequelae as "malaise, poor concentration, nervousness, irritability, emotional lability, and depression" (Gross, 1987) and may itself perpetuate in organic psychosis (Berkow & Fletcher, 1987, p. 935).

Though tryptophan is found in many food substances, it had been routinely available for many years (until the Federal Food and Drug Administration issued a cease-and-desist order in March 1990) in concentrated form as an over-the-counter dietary supplement in health food stores (where it was frequently billed as "nature's tranquilizer"). Tryptophan is also included in several pharmacological preparations intended as dietary supplements for recovering alcoholics and cocaine addicts whose substance abuse has impaired the capacity of their bodies to metabolize niacin. As if to provide a clinical extension, Morand, Young & Ervin (1983) administered oral tryptophan (or a placebo) to a sample of male schizophrenics who had been convicted of violent crimes, with the expected results, but without inquiry into the etiology of the violent behavior of which their subjects had been convicted.[10]

Lithium in the Water Supply?

Lithium is a naturally occurring (rather than synthesized) chemical "element" whose psychoactive properties have been known since the 1870s (Olfson, 1987). Because its principal action tends to calm or tranquilize manic or impulsive behavior, in precise chemical interaction with carbon dioxide it has become (as lithium carbonate) the medication-of-choice in the treatment of manic-depressive schizophrenia (Feldman & Quenzer, 1984, pp. 395–397).

Since lithium *not* in precise combination with carbon dioxide is a natural substance, it is transportable through natural means, such as wind and rain. Thus, University of Texas medical epidemiologists Dawson, Moore & McGanity (1972) studied the level of lithium (apparently released into the air as a by-product of petroleum production) in the water supplies of 200 Texas counties (induced "naturally" through rainfall, rather than added artificially in the manner of fluoridation) in relation to state psychiatric hospital admissions, suicides, and homicides. They found that the higher the rate of naturally transported lithium in the water supply, the lower the rate of homicide as well as of suicide and psychiatric hospital admissions; and, in what must surely be interpreted as an Orwellian proposal, they recommended that "any community should derive prophylactic benefit from lithium ingestion with respect to . . . homicidal tendencies." A scenario of that very sort indeed became the nub of the late physician-novelist Walker Percy's 1987 *The Thanatos Syndrome.* Since heavy concentrations of lithium (or what might be called "overdoses") induce a variety of organically-based psychiatric disorders (Hartman, 1988, pp. 210–211), particular care must be exercised so that concentrations reach "therapeutic" but not "toxic" levels.

Because lithium is a naturally occurring substance and thus differs from other psychoactive substances "created" in pharmacological laboratories, its introduction in precisely controlled concentrations into the water supply of jails, prisons, and mental hospitals may present a different set of legal issues than those which surround the right to refuse psychoactive medication. Similarly, the addition of a dietary supplement like tryptophan to the fare in such facilities may not quite violate that right.

Less Intrusive Dietary Manipulation

There are other naturally occurring substances that can be utilized so as to yield reduction in violence in prison or community settings. At what is surely the least "intrusive" level, Schoenthaler (1982, 1983 a-*d*) has rather convincingly demonstrated that aggressive behavior can be reduced among institutionalized juvenile delinquents, including repetitive violent offenders, as a direct result of the simple dietary manipulation of reducing intake in refined sugar (primarily by substituting unsweetened orange juice for sugar-laden soda and/or fruit for heavily processed snack foods;).[11] One might presume that the addition of orange juice to the menu of correctional and psychiatric institutions, even when coupled with the simultaneous subtraction of soda, would engender fewer objections from civil libertarians than the lithiumization of the water supply or the addition of tryptophan as a ingredient in food preparation, but one cannot be sanguine about the reactions of the soda and candy bar manufacturers.

Paradigm Shift: New Knowledge, New Skills

The body of knowledge and skill marshaled either in the control of neurogenic violence by means of advanced neurosurgery or in the control of impulsivity through cognitive rehabilitation regimens are not commonly available in correctional facilities; nor, for that matter, is it likely that that knowledge and those skills will become commonly available in most public mental hospitals until the paradigm shift courses its way through the mental health system.

Whatever the specific mechanism and whatever the setting, the general direction is clear — viz., that techniques for the management of neurogenic propensities to violence should pivot on strategies for control that marshal the "nearly logarithmic" advances in neuropsychiatry, neurochemistry, and even neurosurgery. And, against the offender's right not to have his body intruded upon against his will, whether by water laced with lithium or by surgical implants into brain tissue, must be balanced, as Monahan (1981) suggested, his next victim's right not to become his next victim.

Conclusion

It has been observed that the standard techniques used to gather data in mental health census surveys do not yield information about neurogenic mental disorders, the identification of which requires detailed neuropsychiatric and/or neuropsychological examination. At best, survey data or even data from psychometric instruments like the MMPI can provide information about the incidence of symptoms like mania, psychopathic deviation, or schizophrenia which may be *secondary* manifestations associated with neurogenic mental disorder.

Alone among the several mental health surveys reviewed in Chapter 2, Pasamanick's (1962) study provided data on organic mental disorder as a distinct category, with a prevalence rate in the general population of only 0.14%. Pasamanick's data derived from "thorough clinical and laboratory evaluations at the Johns Hopkins Hospital," utilizing methods of assessment that were scientifically sound for their time. Since significantly more advanced methods of assessment are now available, it is virtually certain that that ratio represents an underestimate by current scientific standards. Even when the rate of "false negatives" by standard neurological examination found by Cohen, Buonanno, Keck, Finklestein & Benes (1988) is applied to Pasamanick's inventoried prevalence, however, the "adjusted" prevalence rate is no higher than

0.4%., or approximately half that for schizophrenia cited in the NIMH Catchment Area studies (Burke & Regier, 1988).

Though a number of studies have been conducted on groups of offenders for whom the base rate for violence is almost certainly higher than in the general population, and since at minimum correlative association between organic mental disorder and violent behavior has been reasonably well established, one may reasonably infer that the incidence of organic mental disorder in the correctional population is higher than in the general population. But the issue of *how much higher* — i.e., whether by a factor of four, as extrapolation of the Whitman, Coleman, Patmon, Desai, Cohen & King (1984) data might suggest; at 60% of all cases, as the Howard (1984) data might suggest; or on the order of 90% of all cases, as the Yeudall & Fromm-Auch (1979) data might suggest — remains a matter of speculation.

Among the less unreasonable modes of speculation, one might syllabicate the Yeudall & Fromm-Auch (1979) proportions in accordance with the known distribution of prisoners by offense category. Thus, Yeudall & Fromm-Auch found clear evidence of neuropathology in 94% of the homicide offenders they examined, and homicide offenders represent 12.3% of all incarcerated offenders (Flanagan & Jamieson, 1988, p. 494); in 96% of the sex offenders they examined, and sex offenders represent 6.3% of all incarcerated offenders; and in 89% of the assault offenders they examined, and assault offenders represent 7.7% of all incarcerated offenders. The appropriate syllabications and extrapolation would suggest that *neuropathology is to be found in 24% of all incarcerated offenders*, even under the assumption that offenders incarcerated for crimes other than these show a zero incidence of neuropathology. At the very least, that prospect suggests that neuropsychological examination should become a routine feature of the intake process for newly incarcerated offenders in diagnostic and reception centers operated by correctional systems (Fowles, 1988; Gilandas, Touyz, Beumont & Greenberg, 1984; Kaplan, 1990; Spellacy, 1978).

Notes

1. Since the vast majority of those criminal defendants who are found not guilty by reason of insanity are diagnosed as schizophrenic, the implications for forensic assessment are massive; perhaps also there are massive implications for societal constructs of criminal responsibility.
2. Joseph (1990, p.102) also summarizes the case of Charles Whitman, the "Texas Tower" sniper who killed 14 people and wounded 38 others on the University of Texas campus during a 90 minute firing spree in 1966. Long

before his murders, Whitman had consulted a psychiatrist with complaints of "periodic and uncontrollable violent impulses," achieving neither relief nor even an accurate diagnosis. An autopsy revealed in Whitman a "multiforme tumor the size of a walnut compressing the amygdaloid nucleus."

3.   With particular focus on criminal behavior rather than diagnostic category, Hall & McNinch (1988) have summarized the current state of the evidence that links specific *neuroanatomical* (as distinct from *neurochemical)* deficits, anomalies, and impairments to specific categories of crime.

4.   In part on the basis of his earlier research (Hare, 1979, 1982) on psychopathy and cerebral function, in which he had concluded that dysfunction in the dominant hemisphere was unrelated to psychopathy, Hare, undoubtedly the leading authority worldwide on psychopathy, took exception to Gorenstein's findings. In response, Hare (1984) reported contrary data, utilizing a variety of neuropsychological rather than neurological measures (as had Gorenstein), and concluding "psychopaths are less likely to display symptoms of neurological impairment or dysfunction than are individuals who exhibit some of the features of psychopathy but who fall short of fitting the complete clinical syndrome" (p. 139). That description sounds very like Stoudemire's (1987, pp. 135–135) characterization of *organic personality disorder, pseudo-psychopathic type.* In another study, Hare & McPherson (1984) administered a listening task that required activation of lateralized brain functions to inmates who had been classified as high or low in psychopathy and to control subjects who were presumably crime-free but whose level of psychopathy was not inventoried, finding that "psychopaths are characterized by asymmetric low left-hemisphere arousal." These results were replicated and amplified in a study by Jutai, Hare & Connolly (1987).

Whether brain lateralization (or any other brain anomaly, for that matter) represents a uniform characteristic of those who are properly classified as "fitting the complete clinical syndrome" of the psychopath or only of those who "exhibit some of the features of psychopathy," and should instead more properly be labeled as suffering the pseudopsychopathic variety of organic personality disorder, may be a more salient issue at the conceptual level than at the operational level of correctional management, law enforcement, or crime prevention.

5.   Contrary data on the relationship between neuropathology as verified by advanced imaging techniques and MMPI scores were reported by Ball, Archer, Struve & Hunter (1987) of Eastern Virginia Medical College, who found that abnormal EEG patterns were matched on several MMPI scales, including that for "psychopathic deviation, among adolescent psychiatric inpatients. Similarly, Cullum & Bigler (1988) reported that primary elevations on certain MMPI scales invariably followed head injury among patients resultant in lateralized cerebral dysfunction (verified by CT scan) who were treated at the Health Sciences Center of the University of California, San Diego. The question of whether paper-and-pencil instruments like the MMPI can detect the psychological *sequelae* to neuropathology thus remains moot.

6.   An alternate hypothesis holds that the subculture of violence may not be regionally encapsulated but may instead be time-linked to social factors which foster or discourage violence in the larger society. A body of research, both in the United States and cross-nationally, suggests a relatively high

correlation of deaths by violence (homicide, suicide, traffic fatalities, and other accidents), suggesting that certain periods in societal organization tend to favor violent behavior of a variety of sorts.

Day (1984) found such a correlation over a 30-year period in some 40 nations. In a study of the 50 states and the District of Columbia, Sivak (1983) reported a high congruence between the homicide rate and the rate of traffic fatalities in a single year. In a study conducted at the coroner's office in Cleveland, Hirsch, Rushforth, Ford & Adelson (1973) early observed a confluence in the rate of homicide and suicide in a single Midwestern county in the U.S.

On a national scale, Wilbanks (1982) found both a high congruence between suicide rate and accident rate and a positive correlation between suicide and homicide rates in a sample of 181 regions in the U.S., again in a single year. Hollinger's (1979, 1980) data confirmed Wilbanks' findings, with particular emphasis on mortality among young adults.

And Hollinger & Klemen (1982), in a study which analyzed mortality rates from suicide, homicide, and accident throughout the nation between 1900 and 1975, found that these rates "tend to be parallel over time," a finding they interpreted as "reflecting self-destructive tendencies." Virkkunen (1974) similarly found a high correlation between suicide and homicide over a 15-year period in Finland.

From a radically different perspective and one which perhaps holds major social policy implications, Vigderhous (1975) analyzed the net addition to life expectancy among the developing and developed nations of the world were homicide and suicide to be eliminated as causes of death. Elimination of homicide would add 0.07 years, and elimination of suicide 0.76 years, to mean male life expectancy — but elimination of arteriosclerotic and degenerative heart disease would add 2.71 years.

7. Veneziano (1986) and Garcia & Batey (1988) have reviewed a variety of issues relative to consent to treatment among prisoners and among involuntarily committed mental patients.

8. It is a matter of some interest that the American Psychiatric Association filed an *amicus* brief favoring the position of the state, while the American Psychological Association filed its *amicus* brief on the side of the inmate.

    The position of the American Psychological Association is particularly curious at a time when a vocal segment of its membership had raised a clamor demanding that psychologists be granted the right to prescribe psychoactive medication in their own clinical practices.

    For their part, psychiatrists have stoutly resisted that clamor — and, one says thankfully, with very good reason, for the pace of change produced by the major paradigm shift of which Coyle (1988) has written has been so rapid that even many psychiatrists have found themselves outdated in their knowledge of neuropsychopharmacology, as Rubinson, Asnis & Friedman of the Albert Einstein College of Medicine (1988) suggested in their study of "significant errors" in the diagnosis of depression and the consequent decision not to use somatic treatment.

9. The "clear and imminent danger" principle has been articulated most clearly in court decisions concerning the duty of mental health professionals to warn persons whom they have reason to believe are in danger of becoming

victims of violence, even when such a belief arises during the course of psychotherapeutic transactions whose confidentiality is otherwise protected by law. The key decisions arose in the *Tarasoff* case.

In *Tarasoff v. Regents,* the Supreme Court of California affirmed in 1976 that the psychologist who had treated an emotionally disturbed student at the University of California (who admitted during treatment an intention to slay his former girl friend) had a duty to warn the prospective victim and that this duty extended to the psychiatrist who had supervised the treating psychologist and to the Regents of the University, in whose name both were acting; in a 1980 decision in *Thompson v. County of Alameda,* the same Court articulated "the requirement that there be a readily identifiable victim before a duty to warn can be imposed" (Simon, 1987, p. 309).

Litwack & Schlesinger (1987) have reviewed a number of court decisions that have placed upon mental health professionals at a minimum the *duty to warn* those they have reason to believe are in "imminent danger" of victimization on the basis of information revealed by patients. Such a duty requires that the clinician make a "prediction" of violence, albeit with the overt purpose of defeating that prediction (Hall, 1984).

Renowned legal scholar George Dix (1983) has underscored the capital distinction between an assessment of *clear and imminent* danger to a *particular* prospective victim, as explicated in the *Tarasoff* decision, and a more generalized opinion about the prospect that a particular person, at some future time and under some unspecified set of conditions, *might* perpetrate a violent crime.

As Dix puts it (p. 256): "there is little reliable evidence verifying claims made by some members of the [mental health] profession of predictive skill. Such research as is available concerns mostly long term predictions concerning the conduct of persons without traditional mental illness; this research suggests minimal predictive skill . . . psychiatrists' predictive ability is substantially greater when it is called into play concerning the short-term risk posed by persons whose assaultive tendencies are related to symptoms of identifiable serious mental illness. But claims of predictive skill even in these situations might be acknowledged to rest only upon intuition." It is presumably the matter of short-term risk that guided the Court's thinking in *Washington v. Harper.*

But the "clear danger" issue had been broadened by the Court in another landmark case that dealt with the prediction of violence not in the immediate future or against a specific prospective victim.

Instead, in *Barefoot v. Estelle,* 1983, a case which challenged capital punishment, the U.S. Supreme Court upheld the Constitutional permissibility of the prosecution's use of expert psychiatric testimony that plaintiff (who had slain a police officer, apparently with premeditation and careful deliberation) would continue to behave in homicidally violent ways unless he was *executed,* despite a dissenting *amicus* brief submitted by the American Psychiatric Association, recounting an earlier Task Force Report (1974) on the assessment of violence, which had warned: "The state of the art regarding predictions of violence is very unsatisfactory. The ability of psychiatrists or any other professionals to reliably predict future violence is unproved." Incredibly, the Court also held that such expert testimony "need not be based on personal examination of the defendant and may be given in response to hypothetical questions" (Amnesty International, 1987, pp. 217–218).

10.   Protein found in corn is deficient in tryptophan, so that "dietary niacin deficiency is common in areas of the world where corn is a dietary staple." Thus, Mawson & Jacobs (1978) studied the relationship between annual consumption of corn, measured in bushels per capita, and homicide rates across 45 nations of the world; consumption and homicide were found to vary together.

11.   In a study that examined the obverse hypothesis, Rosen, Booth, Bender, McGrath, Sorrell & Drabman (1988) added small amounts of sugar to the diet of preschool and elementary children, reporting "small increases in the children's activity level" (and decrements in cognitive performance among girls) among experimental subjects in relation to controls fed a sugar substitute. Similarly, Kruesi, Rapoport, Cummings & Berg (1987) reported that "duration of aggression against property" was significantly associated with ingestion of sugar, but not of a sugar substitute, among preschool children.

5

Reprise: Estimates of Mental Health Staffing Needs

Implicitly, two questions have guided this excursion: What sorts of mental health problems can be expected among members of correctional populations? What sorts of treatment and treaters are required to address those problems?

The answers, in brief, are respectively: *More than we thought, probably;* and *More than we've got, probably.*

Probable Incidence of Mental Disorder among Prisoners

No one without a feverish brain and an axe to grind could reasonably expect to find among members of a population that is, by definition, deviant a rate of mental disorder that is lower than the rate(s) for relevant segments of the general population. Even when inflected for differences in race and sex, it thus seems entirely unreasonable to expect that the rate of serious mental disorder is less than about 19% *(Figure* 1, Chapter 2), the median figure for fine screen studies both over the course of several years and in the ambitious NIMH Epidemiological Catchment Area studies (Burke & Regier, 1988), which (both because of the precision with which they were designed and their sponsorship) are certain to become the contemporary benchmark in mental health epidemiology.

But even in the absence of enumerative studies (or even studies of reasonably-sized, stratified samples), the fragmentary data drawn from a variety of investigations of prison populations suggest that the rate of mental disorder may be of the magnitude of several times that in the general population.

Prevalence of Pernicious Disorders

Further, given the specific inflections in the demographics of criminally confined populations, the nature of the disorders found in correctional populations are likely to be particularly pernicious:

- Schizophrenia, mania, paranoia, psychopathic deviation in high proportion (the reassembled Megargee-Bohn data, *Figure* 4, Chapter 2);
- Mental deficiency at high prevalence (the Pasamanick and Denkowski & Denkowski data, *Figure* 7, Chapter 2);
- Generalized psychosocial dysfunction even in the absence of clearly-defined symptomatology (the Warheit, Bell, Schwab & Buhl data, *Figure* 2, Chapter 2);
- An extraordinarily high frequency of alcohol and drug use problems (Bureau of the Census studies, *Figure* 10, Chapter 3);
- Neuropsychological deficits (the Bell, Bryant et al., Blackburn, Galski et al., Langevin et al., Whitman et al., and Yeudall & Fromm-Auch studies), psychopharmacological (the Virkkunen et al. reports) and psychoendocrinological (the Bradford & McLean, Boulton, Davis et al., Dabbs et al., Lidberg, Rada et al., and Virkkunen et al. studies) anomalies (described in Chapter 4).

The Effects of Confinement

Psychological disorders that arise as a function of confinement have virtually no analogue among those who are not members of correctional populations; hence, these are virtually ipsative phenomena. Moreover, it is to be anticipated that confinement-specific psychological stress will serve to exacerbate many forms of mental disorder which preexist the experience of incarceration, particularly among those prisoners undergoing a first experience of confinement (Bukstel & Kilmann, 1980; Gunn, 1978; Toch, 1975).

Thus, on the basis of a study of MMPI results among incarcerated offenders at admission and after 115 days in confinement, Bohn & Traub (1986) concluded to "clinical deterioration rather than improvement in adjustment to incarceration" as an early artifact of prisonization. A similar conclusion was reached by MacKenzie & Goodstein (1985) in their investigation of nearly 1300 male offenders:

> Inmates who are new to prison but anticipate serving long sentences experience the greatest stress . . . those new to prison who anticipate serving long terms reported higher levels of stress and lower self-esteem than did those who had already completed long terms. Shortterm subjects new to prison reported less depression and fewer psychosomatic illnesses . . . Those who had received long sentences

and had already served a lengthy time in prison appear to have developed methods of coping with the experience.[1]

Similarly, in their study of methods of coping among inmates of the New York prisons, Toch, Adams & Grant (1989, p. 19) observed a decrease in the number of disciplinary infractions between the first six months and the last six months of an inmate's term, generally on the order of 33% to 50%, though the trend did not obtain for all age groups.

The behavioral manifestation of stress reaction is not infrequently an act of aggression whether, in the present context, directed toward a fellow inmate, toward a member of the prison staff, or inwardly. Such a generalization is supported by studies by Wilmotte & Plat-Mendlewicz (1973) on suicide attempts among prisoners; Levenson (1974) on loss of locus of control as an effect of prisonization; Atlas (1984) and Swett & Hartz (1984) on prison violence; Walkey & Gilmour (1984) on preference for "personal space" and violence among inmates; and Cox, Paulus & McCain (1984), Ekland-Olson (1986), and Ruback & Carr (1984) on prison overcrowding and its consequences.[2]

To the extent that the stress of prisonization interacts with a high incidence of mental disorder and perhaps with biologically-determined deficits in impulse control, the issue of ipsative reactions to confinement are clearly a matter of concern both in prison management and to clinicians who serve offender populations. Thus, one should add to the epidemiologic inventory ipsative disorders that arise from the experience of confinement itself.

Probable Hostility Toward Mental Health Treatment

And one might also add to the mix that members of lower SES groups, if they are treated in the community at all, are typically referred, likely kicking and screaming, for mental health care only as a result of an encounter with police and the courts (as Hollingshead reported; Chapter 2) and are thus not unlikely to greet mental health care providers in correctional settings with a residue of hostility.

Perhaps one should flavor the mix with the generalized lack of impulse control commonly encountered among the criminally deviant, and add to that the characteristic resistance of the psychopathically deviant (whether of the "true" variety identified by Hare or the "pseudo" variety resultant from neuropathology) to mental health treatment of any sort (Meloy, 1988, pp. 333–339).

Probable Incidence in Contrast to the General Population

Comparisons have been made throughout the text between the relative incidence of mental disorder of various sorts found among prisoners in a panoply of studies and that found in the general population in several epidemiological investigations.

In a penultimate recapitulation, the prevalence of various disorders found among prisoners in a range of studies is contrasted in *Figure* 13 with incidence data from the consolidated NIMH Epidemiological Catchment Area studies reported by Burke & Regier (1988), the new benchmark for the general population. It has already been observed that the differences in proportions with which the same disorder is observed among the general population in the NIMH data and among prisoners in the various studies (as assessed by the application of the chi square statistic for comparing proportions drawn from samples of very different sizes) reach statistical significance beyond a probability level of .001 in each case. And, it should be noted, the data recapitulated in *Figure* 13 do *not* reflect the incidence of *neuro*psychological and *neuro*psychiatric disorder observed among offenders, especially violent offenders, in a panoply of investigations, except perhaps as such disorder is pivotal to such conditions as mania, psychopathic deviation, or schizophrenia. Nonetheless, the data in Figure 13 indicate quite clearly that

- The level of mental disorder observed in a variety of investigations among prisoners exceeds that in the general population in every category surveyed in the NIMH Epidemiological Catchment Area studies.

Comparison with Mental Hospital Patients

Perhaps those discrepancies should not surprise us. Prisoners are, by definition, socially deviant; that the incidence of psychiatric deviance among a group already adjudicated as criminally deviant is higher than in the putatively non-deviant (either criminally or psychiatrically) general population may say something about the "clustering" of deviancies.

Pursuit of the notion of the clustering of deviancies leads, perhaps inevitably, to a final comparison – between that group clearly identifiable as criminally deviant (viz., prisoners) and a group clearly identifiable as the psychiatrically deviant segment of the general, or at least of the noncriminal, population (viz., inpatients in public mental hospitals).

Data concerning the extent and character of psychiatric deviance among mental hospital patients are available through the periodic reports issued by the Division of Biometry and Epidemiology of the

Figure 13. Relative Frequency with Which Key Mental Disorders Were Observed among Prisoners and among Respondents in the NIMH Epidemiological Catchment Studies (Burke & Regier, 1988).

Disorder/Source	Prisoners	NIMH Subjects
Alcohol use/dependence		4.7%
Bureau of the Census, 1988	19%	
Cognitive impairment		1.3%
Denkowski & Denkowski, 1986	2%	
Depression		6.3%
Reassembled Megargee-Bohn data	20%	
Drug use/dependence		2.0%
Bureau of the Census, 1988	17%	
Mania		0.5%
Reassembled Megargee-Bohn data	37%	
Obsessive-compulsive disorder		1.5%
Reassembled Megargee-Bohn data	25%	
Psychopathic deviation		0.8%
Reassembled Megargee-Bohn data	58%	
Schizophrenia/Schizophreniform disorder		0.9%
Reassembled Megargee-Bohn data	24%	
Somatization disorder/Hysteria		0.1%
Reassembled Megargee-Bohn data	13%	
Substance abuse disorders, total		6.0%
Bureau of the Census, 1988	54%	

National Institute of Mental Health. A recent analysis reports the diagnosis professionally assigned at admission for the nearly 370,000 patients who are annually admitted to treatment in public mental hospitals (Manderscheid, Witkin, Rosenstein et al., 1985), including the nearly 27,000 (or slightly more than *7%)* who are involuntarily committed as incompetent to stand trial, not guilty by reason of insanity, mentally disordered sex offenders to be confined for treatment in psychiatric facilities, or transferred from prison settings in consequence of florid mental illness (Steadman, Rosenstein, MacAskill & Manderscheid, 1988, p. 94).

Data concerning diagnoses at admission for patients in public mental hospitals (Mandershceid, Witkin, Rosenstein et al., 1985, p. 47) are recapitulated in *Figure* 14 and even more dramatically

Figure 14. Relative Frequency of Diagnosis at Admission to Public Mental Hospitals (Manderscheid et al., 1985) in Relation to Empirically-Derived Estimates of the Incidence of Similar. Disorders among Prisoners.

Disorder/Specification/Source	Prisoners	Inpatients
Affective disorders		6.3%
Depression, Reassembled Megargee-Bohn data	*20%*	
Mania, Reassembled Megargee-Bohn data	*37%*	
Alcohol problems		21.7%
Bureau of the Census, 1988	*19%*	
Anxiety, somatoform, dissociative disorders		13%
Hypochondriasis, Reassembled Megargee-Bohn data	*13%*	
Hysteria, Reassembled Megargee-Bohn data	*13%*	
Psychasthenia, Reassembled Megargee-Bohn data	*25%*	
Cognitive impairment		*Not covered*
Denkowski & Denkowski, 1986	*2%*	
Drug problems		4.8%
Bureau of the Census, 1988	*17%*	
Organic mental disorders		5.3%
Yeudall & Fromm-Auch, 1979, inflected	*24%*	
Personality disorders		5.7%
Psychopathic deviation		
Reassembled Megargee-Bohn data	*58%*	
Schizophrenia and other psychoses		40.0%
Paranoia, Reassembled Megargee-Bohn data	*22%*	
Schizophrenia, Reassembled Megargee-Bohn data	*24%*	
Substance abuse disorders, compounded		*Not covered*
Bureau of the Census, 1988	*54%*	

depicted graphically in *Figure* 15, along with comparable data that indicate the incidence of these disorders (or of disorders within the larger categories employed by NIMH record keeping systems) observed among prisoners. It should be noted that the diagnoses represented in the NIMH categories are independent and summative, while the corresponding incidence among prisoners overlap; data which precisely correspond to the NIMH categories would, among prisoners, relate to the offense-of-record rather than to mental health status.

Figure 15. Graphic Representation of the Relative Frequency of Diagnosis at Admission to Public Mental Hospitals (Manderscheid et al., 1985) in Relation to Empirically-Derived Estimates of the Incidence of Similar Disorders among Prisoners.

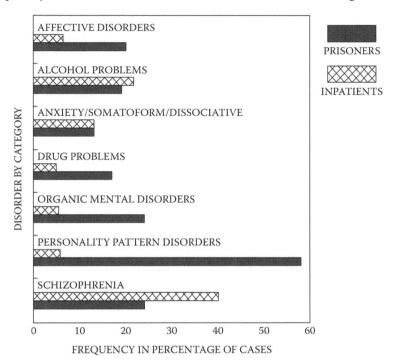

Calculation of the Yates-corrected chi square statistic to test the significance of the difference between the proportions in *Figure* 14 again yields large values, with each comparison significant at a probability of .001 or beyond, except in the cases of schizophrenia, in which the resultant chi square reaches significance at p =.02; alcohol problems, in which the test fails of significance; and the broad category "anxiety, somatoform, and dissociative disorders," in which the difference is null.

Further, with the exception of schizophrenia, the direction of these differences falls toward the incidence observed among prisoners. To follow the NIMH diagnostic categories:

• There is a significantly higher incidence of psychometrically inventoried depression among prisoners than of diagnoses of all *affective disorders* combined among mental hospital patients.

- There is no significant difference between the incidence of *alcohol problems* among prisoners and the frequency of this diagnosis among mental hospital patients.
- There is no significant difference between the relative frequency of diagnoses in the *anxiety, somatoform, and dissociative disorder category* among mental hospital patients and the incidence of psychometrically inventoried hypochondriasis or hysteria (two disorders which specify the larger category) among prisoners; in the case of psychasthenia (obsessive- compulsiveness), the incidence among prisoners for this single disorder is nearly double the frequency of diagnosis for all disorders in this compound category combined among mental hospital patients.
- There is a significantly higher incidence of *drug problems* among prisoners than the frequency of this diagnosis among mental hospital patients.
- There is a significantly higher incidence of *organic mental disorder* among prisoners than the frequency of this diagnosis among mental hospital patients.
- There is a significantly higher incidence of *personality disorder* (specifically, of psychopathic deviation) among prisoners than the frequency of this diagnosis among mental hospital patients.
- However, there is a significantly higher relative frequency of the diagnosis of *schizophrenia* among mental patients than the psychometrically inventoried incidence of this disorder among prisoners.

When one adds to the mix that 100% of the prisoners but only 7% of the mental hospital patients have committed criminal acts for which they have been prosecuted, the clustering of deviancies becomes rather clear.

The Right to "Treatment"and to "Care"

In upholding the decisions of Mr. Justice Frank Johnson in the historic *Wyatt* and *Donaldson* cases, the U.S. Supreme Court declared unequivocally that patients in mental hospitals have an absolute right to treatment and that to confine patients in the absence of treatment in effect constitutes involuntary imprisonment, in violation of Constitutional guarantees against deprivation of liberty without due process (Golann & Fremouw, 1978, pp. 129–185).

That right does not necessarily extend to prisoners, except perhaps to those transferred to mental hospitals from correctional facilities in consequence of florid psychiatric symptomatology (and to those "mentally disordered" sex offenders judicially confined for treatment in such hospitals rather than in correctional settings).

Nonetheless, to the extent that "care" is distinguishable from "treatment," the right of the prisoner to professional mental health intervention of the "care" variety has been established in several Federal court decisions through the level of the U.S. Supreme Court.

The Right of Prisoners to Medical Treatment

Under a variety of Supreme Court decisions, most clearly articulated in *Estelle v. Gamble,* the right of prisoners to *medical* treatment has been rather firmly established, and the failure of correctional administrators to provided treatment has been labeled "deliberate indifference," Constitutionally impermissible under the Eighth Amendment. According to legal scholar Connie Mayer (1990, pp. 2–3):

> The Supreme Court held in *Estelle v. Gamble* that the government's failure to provide adequate medical care for those whom it is punishing by incarceration would result in unnecessary pain and suffering [contrary to the provisions of] the Eighth Amendment to the Constitution which [prohibits] cruel and unusual punishment.

The Right of Prisoners to Mental Health "Care"

To the extent that mental health "care" is distinguishable from mental health "treatment," the right to of prisoners to such care has been judicially determined.

In the landmark *Pugh v. Locke* decision of 1976, upheld by the Supreme Court contemporaneously with *Estelle v. Gamble* (and under the terms of which the prisons of some 30 other states have been reformed by direction of the Federal courts), Mr. Justice Johnson established the right of prisoners to sanitary and "humane" living conditions, to "meaningful programs," to "mental health care," and to a variety of other services.[3]

In an appendix to the *Pugh* decision entitled *Minimum Constitutional Standards for Inmates of Alabama Penal System,* Mr. Johnson ordered that there should be routine provision for identification of "those inmates who, by reason of psychological disturbance or mental retardation require care in facilities designed for such persons" and for the transfer of prisoners thus identified to such (presumably forensic) psychiatric installations. But he also ordered that (with emphases added)

> The defendants [i.e., the state and its prison administration] shall identify those inmates who require *mental health care within the institution and make arrangements for such care.*

113

The *Pugh* decision, then, required both that a mental health census be undertaken for the purpose of identifying inmates in need of mental health care *and* that such care, apparently for disorders which do *not* require psychiatric hospitalization, be provided *in situ* within prison facilities. Since Mr. Johnson made a distinction between those prisoners who were to be transferred to psychiatric hospitals and those for whom "care" was to be provided within prison facilities, the closest analogue to such "care" in the world outside prison walls may be the type of *outpatient* treatment routinely available to the general population through community mental health centers. From the judicial perspective, then, "treatment" appears to be that form of professional intervention provided in psychiatric hospitals, while "care" is that form of intervention to be provided *in situ* for prisoners whose disorders are not severe enough to warrant hospitalization.

In her analysis of Federal decisions over some two decades, Mayer (pp. 3, 9–10) opines that the general trend in decisions in Federal courts (thus far, principally below the level of the Supreme Court) has been toward further clarifying a "right" to mental health care (if not yet quite a right to treatment) for prisoners with mental disorders that rise to a certain level of severity, although that level remains vaguely defined:

> Thus, *Estelle v. Gamble* established an inmate's Eighth Amendment right to treatment for serious physical disorders. Since *Estelle* was decided, there has been a general consensus among courts that there is no logical distinction between the right to medical care for physical ills and the right to mental health care for psychological or psychiatric impairments. Therefore, the deliberate indifference standard has been held to apply to serious mental disorders . . . [But] courts have held that an inmate's statement that he was depressed does not require a prison official to whom the statement was made to schedule him for an appointment with a psychologist since mere depression is not a serious medical need . . . On the other hand, *acute* depression, paranoid schizophrenia, and nervous collapse have been identified as disorders sufficiently dramatic to amount to serious medical need . . . courts will very likely defer to the judgment of mental health care professionals in determining whether an inmate has a serious need.

Moreover, Mayer believes that such professional assessments of severity – of, for example, whether such conditions as neurogenic mania are equivalent to such self-limiting mental disorders as caffeine intoxication, which patently do not require professional intervention in an arena in which not all disorders are created equal – may be susceptible to certain biases that have little to do with scientific objectivity, much less correspondence with commonly accepted lexical canons (p. 10): "A system that wishes to limit the number of inmates within its mental health care system could support that limit through expert testimony which would limit the definition of serious mental illness."

Or, more simply: A system that wishes to limit the provision of mental health care to prisoners might simply *not* undertake a mental health census among those currently incarcerated nor conduct mental health evaluations among new admittees, thereby avoiding that "inconvenient knowledge" upon which "deliberate indifference" might be seen to pivot.

Judicially-Imposed Mental Health Staffing Standards

In *Pugh v. Locke,* Justice Johnson ordered implementation in the Alabama prisons of the mental health staffing ratios proposed by the Center for Correctional Psychology at the University of Alabama (Gormally, Brodsky, Clements & Fowler, 1972), even in advance of the mental health census he had directed to be undertaken.[4]

The Pugh v. Locke *Staffing Standards for Prisons*

That report (p. 54) called for what reduces to an overall ratio of one mental health specialist for each 91 inmates — specifically: one bachelor's level mental health technician or correctional counselor for each 135 inmates; one psychologist for each 506 inmates; one social worker for each 578 inmates; one psychiatrist for each 4048 inmates.

Mr. Johnson's ruling in effect held that these personnel were required to provide "mental health care" as a sort of first-line intervention within the prisons themselves, since the most severe cases were to be transferred to appropriate mental hospital facilities.

Since those ratios were proposed in advance of a comprehensive mental health census, it is not entirely clear what rationale drove the computations; but, as has been observed in Chapter 2, Gormally et. al. had reviewed a number of published and unpublished studies reporting the incidence of mental disorders in correctional populations in a wide range from 15% to 95%, with a median of 38% (p. 21), and with no detail provided in respect of the measuring devices from which the ratios were derived. It is probable, then, that the median ratio governed their recommendations.

Applying the *Pugh* standards to the 545,000 adult inmates of state and Federal prisons (Flanagan & Jamieson, 1988, p. 491), one would expect to find nearly 6200 mental health personnel employed in these facilities (4037 correctional counselors or mental health technicians, 1077 psychologists, 942 social workers, 135 psychiatrists). There are no provisions in the *Pugh* standards for neuropsychiatrists, neurologists, or psychiatric nurses.[5,6]

Even so, application of the *Pugh v. Locke* ratios would mean that 6% of the 101,000 personnel employed in Federal and state prisons for adults (Flanagan & Jamieson, 1988, p. 73) should be mental health specialists, or that the ratio between such specialists and the aggregate number of security and administrative personnel should be on the order of 1:16.

In contrast to the 1:91 ratio between prisoners and mental health specialists ordered in *Pugh,* it might be observed that the ratio between security personnel and inmates in Federal and state prisons is 1:5.4 (*Ibid.*).

Inflection by Differential Incidence of Disorder

Moreover, and perhaps inevitably considering the date of the governing decision, the *Pugh* standards do not (and could not) account the "major paradigm shift" in the mental health sciences that distinguished neuropsychiatrist Joseph Coyle (1988) holds occurred in the decade between 1978 and 1988.

If it be the case, even on the basis of fragmentary data, that the familiar psychological disorders like depression and the psychoneuroses are indeed encountered less frequently in the correctional population than in the general population, the *Pugh v. Locke* standard that bachelor's level "correctional counselors" and "mental health technicians" should constitute the first-line mental health care-providers may be less than relevant to the array of mental disorder disproportionately prevalent among the disproportionately male and nonwhite correctional population, especially those of neuropathologic etiology. Are the disorders likely to be encountered differentially in a correctional population likely to be amenable to such care as is likely to be provided by minimally trained, sub- professional staff, especially at a time when even most doctoral level professionals are still ill-informed about anything more pernicious than depression or the psycho- neuroses?

However appropriate the "interminable talking cure" might be for the middle class anxiety neurotic, it seems unreasonable to expect that the same "curative" process can or should be applied to patients whose impulsivity, lack of foresight, and disregard for the consequences of behavior may emerge directly from a brain that has been congenitally or accidentally disordered or damaged as a consequence of prolonged biochemical insult, or, at an even more primitive level, from neuro-chemical anomalies of unknown etiology. In that context, even first-line mental health care cannot proceed in the absence of pivotal input by neuropsychiatrists at a minimum, augmented by neuroendocrinolo-gists, neuropharmacologists, and perhaps neurosurgeons, when per-haps even doctoral level psychologists (or at least those not well versed in the techniques of clinical neuropsychology) will occupy essentially adjunctive and supportive roles in what Coyle (1988) has termed the "more specific and effective therapies" to emerge from the revolution in the neurosciences.

The Wyatt Staffing Standards for Mental Hospitals

In his decisions in *Wyatt* and *Donaldson*, the landmark cases that established the right to treatment among mental patients, also upheld by the U.S. Supreme Court,[7] Mr. Justice Johnson set out a detailed set of standards for the staffing of public mental hospitals.

In these decisions, in contrast to the 1:91 ratio between mental health care-providers and offenders in the prisons ordered in *Pugh,* he ordered in the public mental hospitals what reduces to an overall ratio of one mental health specialist for every two patients — specifically: 2 psychiatrists, 7 psychologists, 14 social workers, 24 mental health technicians, 11 occupational therapists, and 92 psychiatric aides for every 250 patients.

These mental health specialists are to be augmented by four phy-sicians, eighteen nurses, ten orderlies, and a dental hygienist; again, there are no mandatory provisions for neuropsychiatrists, neurologists, or neuropsychologists.

Inequality between Deviancies – at Deep Discounts

We have observed that the *Pugh* mental health staffing standards were imposed by Mr. Justice Johnson *a priori,* in advance of knowledge of the results of the mental health census among prisoners he had ordered.

We have also acknowledged that deviancies are not created equal, that they come in a variety of shapes and sizes, just like mental disorders of various sorts (and felony crimes, for that matter). But the degree of inequality between criminal deviancy and psychiatric deviancy might be empirically gauged by comparing the number of mental health required personnel for the prisons in *Pugh* with those that would be required for these institutions were the *Wyatt* standards applied.

117

To apply the *Wyatt* standards in a meaningful way in prison settings, we should discard the "psychiatric aide" category altogether, assuming that the roles embedded therein could be played effectively by prison security personnel, as Sandhu (1977) has urged. That discarding yields a net of 58 care-givers to 250 care- recipients, thus increasing the ratio from 1:2 to 1:4.

If one contrasts the 1:91 *Pugh* standard (i.e., one mental health specialist for each 91 prisoners) with the inflected *Wyatt* standard we have already discounted by eliminating psychiatric aides (so that the resulting ratio is 1:4, or one mental health specialist for each four care-recipients), the *judicially-determined* "discount rate" between criminal deviancy and psychiatric deviancy appears to be on the order of 95% — that is, application of the *Wyatt* standards as inflected (by eliminating psychiatric aides altogether) would require some 136,000 mental health specialists in the prisons, or approximately 21 times as many as required under the *Pugh* standards — and more by a third than all personnel employed in the prisons combined.

That comparison, of course, represents an exercise in sheer fantasy. It is also grossly inappropriate, for a variety of reasons.

First, Mr. Johnson imposed the *Pugh* ratio *in advance of* the mental health census he had ordered, so that the prospect that significant mental disorder constitutes the rule rather than the exception among imprisoned offenders could not be calculated into the equation. Second, he specifically ordered that those offenders in need of inpatient mental hospitalization for reasons of mental retardation or, one presumes, because of florid symptomatology not controllable outside a medical facility be so transferred. Clearly, then, the *Pugh* standards are intended to apply to institutions whose purpose is *not* to treat psychiatric deviancy, but upon which, in Mr. Johnson's decision, an obligation to provide mental health care *as a health care service in situ* nonetheless devolves.

Third, and most important, the *Wyatt* standards are intended to apply to institutions whose *sole* purpose is the treatment of psychiatric deviancy and in which the rate of mental disorder among inmates may comfortably be assumed to be 100%. One might presume that each of the inmates of those institutions (or at least each of the 93% who have not been involuntarily committed) is anxious for mental health treatment, although many clinicians who have served in public mental hospitals might be unwilling to ascribe such an assiduous desire universally among mental patients, however (Beck & Golowka, 1988). But the same assumption about a universal desire for treatment cannot be made of confined offenders — for a variety of reasons ranging from the ego- syntonic character of certain disorders prevalent in correctional populations (e.g., mania, psychopathic deviation) to the typical pathways of referral to mental health treatment among offenders from lower SES groups, who may be expected to regard such treatment as essentially punitive in character; thus, active resistance is likely to be a modal response to the availability of treatment (Halleck, 1987, pp. 162–165).

Inflecting the Wyatt Ratios by Inventoried Disorder

But univocal application of the *Wyatt* standards also yields unrealistically high figures by implying the provision of mental health care for prisoners who, by our own inventory, are not in need of such care, quite apart from their receptiveness or resistance.

As inspection of the reassembled Megargee-Bohn data (*Figure* 4, Chapter 2) suggests, it may be the case that 24% of prison inmates are free of psychometrically inventoried mental disorder, so that only 76% are putatively in need of mental health care. If one further makes the questionable assumption that the 26% of those inmates who are likely classifiable as organically mentally disordered (the Yeudall & Fromm-Auch data, Chapter 4) are subsumed among those with scores above the clinical threshold on such MMPI scales as schizophrenia, mania, or psychopathic deviation,[8] one could reduce the total prison population putatively in need of mental health care to 74%. Similarly, we could presume that the very high proportions of incarcerated offenders with alcohol or drug problems or combinations thereof (Bureau of the Census data; *Figure* 10, Chapter 3) are similarly accounted for by scores on the MMPI scales, individually or in combination, beyond the clinical threshold and thus let the 74% proportion stand. From that figure, however, we should subtract the 2% of inmates found in the Denkowski & Denkowski (1986) study (*Figure* 7, Chapter 2) to be mentally retarded, who, according to *Pugh*, should be transferred from prisons to the appropriate facilities in any event.

Those calculations would leave a residue of 72% of the correctional population who require "mental health care," whether in correctional institutions or otherwise. As we have seen earlier in this chapter, Steadman, Rosenstein, MacAskill & Manderscheid (1988) report that 27,000 of the inpatients admitted annually to public mental hospitals are referred through criminal justice channels. From that total, however, should be subtracted the 15,000 who are referred judicially as incompetent to stand trial, as not guilty by reason of insanity, or as mentally disordered sex offenders who are to be treated in hospitals; that leaves 12,000 transferred *from* prison facilities, presumably as a consequence of mental disorder of sufficient severity that treatment outside a hospital setting is not appropriate. And that 12,000 represents 2% of the total prison population, so that we should further reduce our already-inflected residue by an additional 2%, leaving 70% of the total as our target population putatively in need of what Bush (1983) has called "treatment for the guilty" *in situ.*

If one were to assume that the level of mental disorder in that residue were *not* of sufficient severity to warrant transfer to inpatient psychiatric hospitalization, application of *Wyatt* standards we have already heavily discounted to the inmate population in Federal and state correctional institutions for adults *thus reduced* would require an aggregate mental health staff in the prisons of 95,000 — or nearly equal to the current total roster of all prison employees combined and 15 times greater than that projected by *Pugh v. Locke* standards.

If one assumes that half of all those prisoners putatively in need of mental health care are so resistant as to reject such care out of hand (a not altogether unreasonable assumption), application of the modified *Wyatt* standards would require an aggregate mental health staff on the order of 47,500, or nearly half the total roster of all prison employees and some eight times greater than those required under *Pugh.*

These calculations are clearly an exercise in the sheerest sort of perverse fantasy. Let's, instead, take the toughest of the tough minded interpretations of the data we have reviewed and make the assumption that the rate of mental disorder among incarcerated offenders is *no greater* than that found in "fine screen" studies or in the new benchmark NIMH studies of mental health and illness in the general population. Application of the *Wyatt* standards to a mere 19% of the prison population would require a cadre of nearly 26,000 mental health specialists, a figure that exceeds the figure required under *Pugh* by four-fold — so that the discount rate between deviancies reduces to only 75%.

We can take our pick among and between these discount rates; however deviancies may cluster, it is clear that criminal and not psychiatric deviancy governs, even when clustered deviancies are, in the parlance of the mental health professions, comorbid.

Staffing Standards in Community Mental Health Centers

Another comparison might be made, contrasting mental health staffing ratios judicially imposed in prisons and in public mental hospitals with those to be met by outpatient mental health centers designed to provide "first-line" mental health care to the general population; since these centers also frequently function as a referral source to inpatient psychiatric hospitalization, there is a strong analogue with mental health services in prisons.

Although the Joint Commission on Accreditation of Hospitals affiliated with the American Medical Association has published a *Consolidated Standards Manual for Child, Adolescent, and Adult Psychiatric, Alcoholism, and Drug Abuse Facilities* (1983) by which such outpatient facilities are judged, numerical ratios have been avoided therein — for all facilities, including both hospitals and outpatient centers. Instead, the Standards governing staff (p. 18) are stated in very general terms (with emphases added):

> 4.2. The facility shall have enough appropriately qualified health care professional, administrative, and support staff available to adequately assess and address the *identified clinical needs* of patients.
>
> 4.2.1 Appropriately qualified professional staff may include qualified psychiatrists and other physicians, clinical psychologists, social workers, substance abuse workers, psychiatric nurses, and other health care professionals *in numbers and variety appropriate to the services offered by the facility.*
>
> 4.2.2 When appropriate qualified professional staff members are not available as needed on a full-time basis, arrangements shall be made to obtain sufficient services on an attending, continuing consultative, or part-time basis.

Those standards are, of course, to be read within an operational context which includes other mental health facilities (e.g., psychiatric wards or outpatient clinics operated by general medical and surgical hospitals) and service providers (e.g., private practitioners in the mental health professions) within each community mental health catchment area.[9,10] They are thus pertinent to the matter of mental health services for offenders under the supervision of probation authorities but not for those incarcerated in prison facilities.

Notes

1. Wormith (1984), who found that self-esteem during imprisonment varied inversely with post-release recidivism, would clearly disagree – and doubtless

plan a prison program so as to lower the self-esteem of inmates. However that may be, Mabli (1985) found clear evidence of a major increase in stress among both male and female Federal prisoners immediately prior to release.
2.   Flanagan & Jamieson (1988, p. 501) report that, collectively, state prisons operate at 112% capacity on a nationwide basis. California leads the nation, at 153% capacity, followed by Pennsylvania at 150%; at the other end of the spectrum, New Mexico's prisons operate at 77% of capacity. That there are wide variations in the ratio between population and provision of prison facilities across the various states is also a matter of interest; for example, North Carolina, with a population of 6.5 million, has nearly as many prison beds as Ohio, with a population of 11 million (Bureau of the Census, 1989, p. 24). One must presume such factors are implicitly or explicitly weighed during sentencing decisions.
3.   The *Wyatt* decisions (*Wyatt v. Stickney, Wyatt v. Alderholt, Wyatt v. Hardin*) and those in attendant cases (*Donaldson v. O'Connor, O'Connor v. Donaldson*) through the level of the Supreme Court are reproduced in their entirety by Golann & Fremouw (1976). Mr. Justice Johnson's decision in *Pugh v. Locke* is reproduced in *406 Federal Supplement 318*, 1976, pp. 332–337. Golann & Fremouw review in detail a series of cases involving the rights of mental patients, including those confined by judicial action following prosecution for criminal behavior. Among their volume's many interesting features are "eyewitness" accounts by Stonewall B. Stickney, Alabama's commissioner of mental health and therefore the chief executive officer for the state's public psychiatric hospitals during the prosecution of the landmark cases that established, at the level of the U.S. Supreme Court, the rights of mental patients. Similarly, an eyewitness account of his personal role in shaping and prosecuting *Pugh v. Locke* is provided by distinguished psychologist Raymond Fowler (1976, 1988).
4.   Fowler (1988) has recounted in detail the procedures mounted in the implementation of the judicially ordered survey of the psychological "needs" of Alabama's prisoners, which involved assembling of a team of psychologists from around the country in a "crash" program to meet Mr. Johnson's deadlines.
5.   Pallone & LaRosa (1979) and Pallone, Hennessy & LaRosa (1980) further discuss the *Pugh v. Locke* staffing ratios in relation to the standards proposed by such professional groups as the American Correctional Association.
6.   Case law continues to develop in Federal courts, sometimes through contradictory opinions that may ultimately be resolved at the level of the Supreme Court. Thus, according to Mayer (1990, pp. 23–24), the Federal District Court for New Mexico ruled in *Doran v. Anaya* (1986), that that state's plan to reduce its mental health specialist to prisoner ratio from 1:60 to 1:94 "would reduce services so dramatically that psychiatric needs of prisoners would go unmet, thereby inflicting unnecessary pain and suffering [and] adversely affect the minimum constitutional rights of the inmates." Yet, in a vastly incongruent ruling, the Federal District Court for the Eastern District of Pennsylvania found, in *Peterkin v. Jeffes*, that the provision of mental health specialists in two prisons in that state on a ratio of 1:139 did *not* violate minimal Constitutional standards *(Ibid.,* pp. 32–33). Mayer observes: "Most courts require some access to on-site psychiatric care

and generally require that staff be adequately trained to identify and assess the psychiatric needs of inmates. The rest of the numbers game, however, offers little in the way of guidelines for what is constitutionally mandated . . . the recent cases seem to turn importantly on the adequacy of staffing and quality of the contacts with inmates."

7. Brown & Smith (1988) reviewed the compliance of the various states with the Federal Mental Health Systems Act of 1980 which followed the *Wyatt* decisions, with a particular focus on implementation of the rights of patients, concluding that "the only significant predictor is the extent to which each state followed the typical time path of de-institutionalization" — that is, only when the inpatient populations in mental hospitals *declined* did the states implement the rights of the resultant smaller cadre of inpatients served. The investigators comment (pp. 162, 164): "The actions taken by individual states [to implement the rights of mental patients] do not appear to be related to their overall approach to social problems."

8. That this assumption is not entirely warranted is attested by the conflicting results in the studies by Langevin et al. (1987) on offenders and Ball et al. (1987) and Cullum & Bigler (1988) on non-offenders who had suffered medically-verified neuropathologic injury, reviewed in Chapter 4. Nonetheless, Ruff, Ayers & Templer (1977) have argued that certain scale elevations on the MMPI constitute quite gross screens for organic mental disorder.

9. Because community mental health centers have the obligation to provide what might be construed as "emergency" mental health services for acute episodes and because emergency treatment thus necessarily assumes a greater salience than precise diagnosis in such facilities, the category "diagnosis deferred" tends to be reported with substantial frequency in such installations, so that attempts to inventory the character of disorder treated tend to lack precision. Thus, in his survey of patient care episodes in outpatient mental health facilities, Morton Kramer (1977, p. 18) of the Johns Hopkins School of Hygiene and Public Health reported that 58% of the patient care episodes among males and 56% among females lacked precise diagnoses. Among the cases in which a (more or less) firm diagnosis was reported, schizophrenia was reported as the principal disorder among males, at 14%, followed by depressive and alcohol disorders, at 9% each, mental retardation at 4%, organic brain syndromes and drug disorders at 3% each, and psychoses other than schizophrenia at 1%. Among females, schizophrenia and depressive disorders were the leading disorders treated, at 17% each, with each of the other categories represented either by 1% or 2% of the patient care episodes.

10. Like the standards enunciated by JCAH, those adopted by the American Bar Association (1989) as its *Criminal Justice Mental Health Standards* are similarly rather general and non-specific. Though the ABA observed that "No informed observer can fail to reflect upon the prevalence of significant mental abnormalities exhibited by detainees, defendants, and convicts" (p. xvi) and specifically noted the disproportionate incidence of mental illness in relation to race ("Many underprivileged persons caught up in the criminal process suffer the further disadvantages of mental affliction or retardation"), its recommendations are essentially hortatory rather and

prescriptive, in general conforming to the contours of established and emergent case law.

Thus, without essaying to define how it construes "adequacy," Standard 7-10.2 (p. 510) holds that: "Correctional facilities should provide a range of mental health and mental retardation services for prisoners and should have adequately trained personnel readily available to provide such services." Similarly, in the case of the severely afflicted, the ABA recommends (*Idem*) that "Prisoners who require mental health treatment or mental retardation habitation not available in the correctional facility should be transferred to a mental health or mental retardation facility, preferably under the supervision of the jurisdiction's department of mental health or mental retardation."

6

After-Words: Parables of Convenient Ignorance and Casual Indifference

This exercise has focussed on incarcerated offenders, who have been portrayed, to borrow Rogers' (1987, p. 845) telling phrase, as "impaired yet morally repugnant individuals." Though psychiatric and criminal deviancies may cluster in these offenders, the latter essentially govern the treatment accorded them following conviction and imprisonment, with the former largely suppressed or ignored. That may or may not be as it should be; in some large measure, our societal willingness to ignore the former is linked to whether we are willing to ignore dental abscess, influenza, or pneumonia in an offender population because (to borrow Leo Srole's phrasing) these deviancies from an asymptomatic state of wellness are as irrelevant to the punishment for past criminal behavior and the deterrence of future criminal behavior as is mental disorder — or to regard some forms of physical and mental illness as "not serious enough" to warrant professional intervention.

A Demurrer about Causality

Beyond reviewing data on the relative infrequence of apprehension and conviction (Chapter 2), this volume has had little to say about those who, though convicted, have been placed on probation and nothing at all to say about those who commit crimes but are not apprehended, convicted, and confined to correctional institutions. To that extent, it affirmatively *demurs* to any position whatsoever on a causal relationship between mental disorder and criminal behavior. It may be the case that there obtains such a relationship; but, if so, one will never find it by considering data having to do with what is probably only a minor proportion of all those who commit criminal offenses.

125

Information about the probable relative incidence of mental disorder among prisoners is thus very likely not in the least useful to a theory of criminogenesis. Given markedly low rates of apprehension and conviction, there is every reason to believe that those incarcerated in correctional facilities are *not* representative of those who commit criminal offenses. Only were there reasonable congruence between those who commit crimes and those who are imprisoned could one even begin to interpret data on mental disorder among incarcerated offenders in any fashion that approximates "causation." If there is such congruence, we will never know it from studies of imprisoned offenders only; and, in "real world" terms, we are unlikely ever to develop a data base that accurately represents those who commit crimes but are not apprehended and punished therefor.

But, at some fundamental level, wonder about this: If it were the case that mental disorder is in no dependable way associated with criminal behavior, at least correlatively, would it not follow that there should be no greater rate of such disorder among incarcerated offenders than among the non-offender general population? And if the data, even the fragmentary data, are contrary to that expectation, hadn't one better begin searching for a cocked hat large enough to serve as a receptacle for the discarding of cherished beliefs?

Even more primitively, worry about the emerging evidence on the neurogenesis of violent crime, about the disproportionate incidence of neurogenic mental disorder among the poor and the nonwhite, and especially about the utter failure of societal institutions to identify and to treat neuropsychological and neuropsychiatric anomalies, especially among the poor and the nonwhite, before they ever "mature" into criminal behavior; or even to make mental health services available, accessible, and attractive long before that traumatizing referral by police or the courts. Or, alternately, should we admit that maybe, since the victims in violent crime (neurogenic or not) perpetrated by the poor and the nonwhite are usually themselves poor and nonwhite (O'Brien, 1987), that situation serves the rest of us just fine?

Mental Health Care vs. Correctional Rehabilitation

Contemporaneously with the *Pugh v. Locke* decision, the criminal justice and mental health communities were deeply exercised about mounting evidence of the relative *in*effectiveness of psychosocial rehabilitative regimens in the prisons.

Controversy surrounded publication of a landmark study by sociologist Robert Martinson (1974, amplified by Lipton, Martinson & Wilks [1975] in a more detailed monograph) that concluded that most offender rehabilitation regimens for adult prisoners constitute a colossal waste of professional energy and taxpayers' money. That dire judgment was essentially repeated by Shamsie (1982) in an ambitious review of the research evidence on the effectiveness of similar rehabilitation efforts among juvenile offenders. That the government agency which had sponsored the Martinson study suppressed its release and that it saw the light of day only in trials following the prisoner revolt at the New York state prison at Attica surely piqued the interest of the press. Predictably, members of the professional community committed to rehabilitation as a governing purpose of corrections sought to answer the Martinson judgments (Cullen & Gilbert, 1982; Gendreau & Ross, 1979, 1981; Glaser, 1976, Miller, 1977), often with more heat than light. As Martinson (1976) himself suggested, these responses may have issued from a sense of disbelief that "all the well-intentioned efforts of the psychiatric, psychological, and social service communities, of the medical establishment, of the prisons and the jails, and even of the schools have yielded such disappointing results."

The controversy reached even into the prestigious National Academy of Sciences, which commissioned a blue-ribbon panel to re-analyze the more than 200 studies of rehabilitation effectiveness on which the Lipton, Martinson & Wilks conclusions were based (Sechrest, White & Brown, 1979). Those excruciating reanalyses (Feinberg & Gramsbach, 1979) did little to alter the "gloomy conclusions" reached by Martinson — though in what may have been more a leap of faith than a reasoned scientific judgment, Sechrest, White & Brown, (1979, p. 34) focussed on such issues as flaws in the research design of those studies upon which the "gloomy conclusions" rested: "The quality of the work that has been done . . . militate[s] against any policy reflecting a final pessimism."

Yet another re-analysis of that data base by British researchers completed nearly 20 years after Martinson's initial salvo similarly focused on the adequacy of the research design employed in the studies represented therein, and, like the National Academy of Science review, reluctantly declines to draw any sharp conclusion, whether positive or negative. In Clive Hollin's (1990, pp. 119–120) account:

> The ambiguity in clinical outcome studies has been used in both the United Kingdom and the United States to fuel the doctrine

maintaining that "nothing works"; that is, any attempt at rehabilitation is doomed to failure . . . This research is often quoted by those in favor of therapeutic nihilism . . . [yet] the small number of acceptable studies immediately limits the data base from which any conclusions can be drawn, and the subject matter of these studies allows no conclusions to be made . . .

Nonetheless, sentiment both among policy makers and among correctional administrators has veered sharply in the direction of abandoning rehabilitation as a goal of prison incarceration and toward a definition (or a re-definition, once and for all) of the prison as an institution whose purpose is to deter and to punish, not to rehabilitate — in short, as an institution where wrong-doers are met with their "just deserts" (von Hirsch, 1976, 1985). From that perspective, if psychosocial rehabilitation in the correctional setting is to be justified in terms of social economy, it should not be necessary to resort to recondite modes of data analysis to ferret out whatever small statistical advantages may issue from rehabilitative regimens; rather, those advantages should be massive and clear to justify the additional funding required to support such regimens.

In consequence of such a definition or re-definition, one might expect little attention to be paid to issues like the relative incidence of mental disorder among offenders who had been sentenced to prison *not* for rehabilitation but specifically for deterrence and for punishment, or to arcane questions bearing upon the number and character of mental health care-givers in institutions whose purpose is *not* rehabilitation, the *Pugh* and *Estelle* precedents and Constitutionally impermissible "deliberate indifference" notwithstanding — and perhaps not even pertinent.

Yet even so articulate a spokesman for the "just deserts" point of view as the distinguished legal scholar and criminologist Norval Morris (1974, pp. 14–15) has made the capital distinction between (*a*) mental health care *as a health service* for confined offenders and (*b*) psychosocial rehabilitation applied to those mental disorders thought to be "causative" of criminal behavior:

> "Rehabilitation," whatever it means and whatever the program that allegedly gives it meaning, must cease to be a purpose of the prison sanction. This does *not* mean that the various . . . treatment programs within prisons need to be abandoned; quite the contrary, they need expansion. But it does mean that they must not be seen as *purposive* in the sense that criminals are to be sent

to prison *for* treatment . . . The system is corrupted when we fail to preserve this distinction and this failure pervades the world's prison programs.

Just so. And justly so.

But, from the perspective of verifiable formal mental disorder, the terms of the discussion about punishment vs. rehabilitation seem not so much wrong-headed as wrong-ended. To regard psychological rehabilitation (or dental care, for that matter) as the *purpose* of imprisonment requires a conviction (optimally supported by strong empirical evidence) that criminal behavior is the consequence of mental (or dental) disorder, with perhaps a hint that in nearly all cases the degree of culpability attached to such criminal behavior should be tempered precisely in consequence thereof. There is no body of strong evidence to support such a conviction, and, into the bargain, there is evidence that psychosocial rehabilitation in the prisons is in no reliable manner associated with subsequent reduction in recidivism.

Even so, once we have reason to believe that our prisons are populated by people among whom psychometrically inventoriable formal mental disorder is the *norm* rather than the exception, and in a context in which "deliberate indifference" is Constitutionally impermissible, we are very close to the point at which we need to reconceptualize what a prison *qua institution for deterrence and punishment* is, or should be.

Unless we are prepared to let that son-of-a-bitch bellowing on A Wing suffer with his impacted wisdom tooth, because he didn't exactly get a ticket of admission to A Wing along with his Boy Scout merit badge. If he were out on the street, he could go to a dentist or not; it would be none of our concern. We have restricted his liberty, and justly so. What obligation does that place on us?

It may not even be too far-fetched to set forth the proposition that denial of dental treatment can be construed as both punitive and as deterrent. Indeed, in some proportion of the cases, dental abscess might "mature" into general systemic infection which may prove fatal — in which case, we could confidently predict zero recidivism.

A Parable about Elephants and Giraffes

When I was a wee child, my daddy took me to the National Zoo in Washington's Rock Creek Park. Among the day's features was a visit to the Elephant House. The National Zoo differs from other installations of its genre by keeping not just one or two pachyderms but veritably a whole herd; that's why it needs a whole Elephant House.

Now it came to pass on the day of that visit that some minor renovation was in progress in the cages for giraffes. Accordingly, these animals had been moved to temporary quarters in the Elephant House, while the elephants were apparently wandering elsewhere in the Park. I can't quite remember, but I assume that the elephant keepers had accompanied those animals on their outing, so that the handlers we encountered in the Elephant House were giraffe keepers, but I didn't know that at the time; nonetheless, I associated the distinctive uniform they wore with elephant handlers.

Little children are very trustful. If the thing lives in a place that has a sign that proclaims it's the Elephant House, then of course it must be an elephant. For some time, I insisted to the other kids on the playground that an elephant was a very tall animal, with a long neck, because, you see, if the thing lives in an Elephant House, it must be an elephant. And, of course, their managers must be elephant keepers.

Some mental health professionals are inordinately fond of a measuring procedure called an incomplete sentence blank. A sentence stem is provided; the task of the subject is to supply a predicate.

On the basis of the data we have reviewed, how might we construct an *empirically based* predicate that describes the prison?

It might go something like this: A prison is a place *where people who display a higher incidence of mental disorder than is discerned in the general population and is, in the aggregate, not very different in character or severity from that found among patients in public mental hospitals are sent* to be punished, *because they have committed criminal acts.*

And what predicate might be supplied for the psychiatric hospital? Perhaps: A psychiatric hospital is a place *where people who display mental disorder that is, in the aggregate, not very different in character or severity and not massively higher in prevalence from that found among criminal offenders confined to prisons are sent* to be treated, *because they have not (or at least the 93% of them not referred for admission through criminal justice channels putatively have not) committed criminal acts.*

So: *Who lives in the Elephant House? And why?*

Because deviancies cluster; but some deviancies are more equal than others. And because the way in which the society defines the deviancy dictates differentially how we deal with those who are declared deviant in one way but not the other — as well as the discount rate to be applied to one deviancy but not the other.

Brushing aside the issue of what character of professional staff and of intervention modality might prove "more specific and effective" in

Coyle's (1988) terms in relation to those mental disorders *differentially* inventoried among imprisoned offenders, suppose we found in the prisons the staffing pattern for mental health specialists that *Pugh v. Locke* requires, let alone the fantasy numbers required by the *Wyatt* standards. Could we identify the point at which a prison stops being *merely* a facility for deterrence and "punitive corrections" and is forced to become some other kind of institution, or at which we are forced to re-define the nature of a prison *qua* prison?

That son-of-a-bitch on A Wing is bellowing again, and I don't care whether he's got an impacted wisdom tooth or is hearing Voices or seeing things that aren't there. Let him suffer, because he didn't exactly get a ticket of admissions to A Wing along with his Boy Scout merit badge. If he were out on the street, he could go to a shrink or not; it would be none of our concern. We have restricted his liberty, and justly so. Let the governing deviancy govern.

Perhaps Stephen Vincent Benet said it best: Do not burden us with inconvenient knowledge.

Shrinks, peddle your wares elsewhere, particularly shrinks with bleeding hearts who pose as tough minded, masquerade behind an avalanche of numbers, but try to persuade us to look carefully at what lives in the Elephant House — when we can all read the sign on the door and decode the meaning of the uniforms the keepers wear perfectly clearly.

If we avoid the burden of inconvenient knowledge, we can scarcely be accused of deliberate indifference toward that about which we have avoided knowing.

Just so. Let the governing deviancy govern.

7

General Summary

Though no comprehensive, enumerative mental health census has been undertaken among imprisoned offenders, a wide variety of relevant studies coalesce to provide responsive data. It has been the sense of this monograph that:

- In contrast to an incidence of mental disorder among the general population severe enough to warrant professional attention that, on the basis of discerning studies sponsored by the National Institute of Mental Health, can be said to hover around 19%, it is reasonable to believe that the incidence of psychometrically-inventoried mental disorder among offender populations more nearly approximates 74%. Thus, *it may be the case that the overall prevalence of mental disorder is nearly four times greater among imprisoned offenders than in the general population.*
- Given the demographic differences between the general population and imprisoned offenders (who are disproportionately male, nonwhite, and from the lower socioeconomic strata), the inflected prevalence of mental disorder among offenders seems to resemble that among the relevant reference groups in the general population.
- It is reasonable to believe that the incidence of mental retardation among imprisoned offenders exceeds that in the general population by 50%.
- In contrast to an incidence of alcohol and substance abuse problems in the general population that, also on the basis of NIMH studies, can be said collectively to hover near 7%, data from Bureau of the Census surveys among imprisoned offenders suggests an incidence of alcohol problems on the order of 19%, of drug problems on the order of 17%, and of interactive alcohol drug problems on the order of 54%. Thus, *it is probable that the prevalence of alcohol, drug, and combined alcohol/ drug problems is between five and eight times greater among imprisoned offenders than in the general population.*
- Substantial research evidence, much of it conducted utilizing correctional populations, has now demonstrated a possible neurogenic basis for criminal violence. Some studies suggest a very high incidence of neuropathology among violent offenders inflected by type of crime.

When the appropriate syllabications are made with respect to the proportion of imprisoned offenders incarcerated for specific crimes to which a correlative association with neuropathology has been demonstrated, *it is reasonable to believe that neuropathology is to be found in 24% of all imprisoned offenders.* That incidence is more than four times greater than the incidence of organic mental disorder among inpatients in public psychiatric hospitals and some 1700 times as great as that found in the only study (Pasamanick, 1962) that has essayed to detect this class of disorder in the general population by reasonably sophisticated methods of examination. The evidence on whether significant neuropathology is subsumed into clinically elevated scores on such differential diagnostic instruments as the Minnesota Multiphasic Personality Inventory remains mixed; it may be the case that some, all, or none of the cases of neuropathology are detectable thereby.

• In comparison to patients admitted to public mental hospitals, the prevalence of affective disorders is perhaps three times as great among imprisoned offenders; of drug problems, four times as great; of organic mental disorders, four and a half times as great; of personality disorders, eleven times as great. The prevalence of schizophrenia is more than half again greater among mental hospital patients than among imprisoned offenders; there are no significant differences in alcohol problems or neurotic anxiety disorders between these populations.

From such an inventory flow a number of implications for mental health staffing and for the character of mental health care to be provided, under terms of the *Pugh v. Locke* decision, to imprisoned offenders *in situ:*

• Given a set of circumstances in which psychometrically-inventoried mental disorder characterizes a substantial majority of the prison population, it is likely that the standards for mental health care in the prison judicially imposed in *Pugh v. Locke* are inadequate, both in terms of ratios between care-givers and care-recipients and in terms of the character of care-givers professionally prepared to provide professional service to offenders whose mental disorders are those characteristically associated with male, nonwhite, and lower socioeconomic status populations (i.e., those disorders more likely to arise neurogenically).
• Application of standards for mental health care designed for patients in mental hospitals (another group of confined citizens with a high incidence of mental disorder), as judicially imposed in the *Wyatt* decisions, rather than those for such care in prison facilities would enrich the ratio between care-givers and care-recipients in correctional facilities by more than 20 times.
• Given the explosion of knowledge in the neurosciences of the recent past with a resultant "major paradigm shift" in the mental health

sciences, it is clear that the character of mental health care in correctional facilities must be enriched by the unique contributions of neuropsychiatry and neuropsychology. There is already at hand sufficient evidence to warrant addition of comprehensive neuropsychological examination to the classification process at diagnostic and reception centers operated by correctional systems. Serious consideration should be given to the addition of cognitive rehabilitation, neurosurgery, and the non-therapeutic use of psychopharmacological agents as routine features of mental health care in correctional institutions.

No brief has been argued in this volume about whether criminal behavior is a by-product of mental disorder, nor whether psychosocial rehabilitation intended to reduce recidivism should represent the governing purpose of imprisonment. Instead, this volume has assembled data bearing on the relative incidence of mental disorder among imprisoned criminal offenders, without any assumption of a causal relationship between such disorder and crime, but in the firm and fixed belief that the design and implementation of Constitutionally-required *health care* services — as such services are distinguishable both from rehabilitation and from "treatment" — for imprisoned offenders cannot realistically proceed in the absence of such an inventory.

Nor has this volume advanced the naive argument that those offenders classifiable as mentally disordered are themselves eager for mental health treatment, even though the current state of the law surely argues that they are *entitled* to such treatment; or the equally naive argument that there currently obtains an armamentarium of clinical treatment modalities predictably effective both in the reduction of resistance and in the remediation of mental disorder. Because the labels we apply in some large measure dictate behavior, both on the part of those who manage the correctional enterprise and on the part of the offender, one could hardly expect otherwise. To inflect the label appropriately and to develop those "more specific and effective therapies" of which Coyle (1988) has spoken deserve to become major entries on the future agenda for the management of prisons.

Instead, the terms of this inquiry have been essentially syllogistically linear:

- The evidence suggests that some very large proportion of imprisoned offenders display such mental disorder as is classifiable according to the current lexicon which guides the mental health sciences (that is, the American Psychiatric Association's *Diagnostic and Statistical Manual*).

- The current state of the law leads to no other conclusion that they should be accorded mental health care. One may, therefore, conclude both to *need* and to *presumptive entitlement.*

- In common with many other prospective care-recipients who are both mentally disordered and presumptively entitled but are neither criminal nor imprisoned, one may expect that some high proportion of mentally disordered prisoners will not only not welcome such mental health care but may be highly resistant thereto. One can*not,* therefore, conclude to a *want* that corresponds to an inventoried need.

- Moreover, there is little reason to believe that those methods of intervention developed in the mental health professions to serve clients who "want" mental health services (that is, principally those who perceive their disorders as ego-dystonic) are applicable without modification to other clients, whether guilty of criminal behavior or not and whether punitively incarcerated or not.

- To address the question of resistance and to develop those methods of intervention particularly effective in mental health care for resistant, confined clients constitute prime entries on an agenda that deserves to be constructed. But construction of that agenda cannot commence without an appraisal of "need" through a rational approximation to an epidemiologic inventory of mental disorder among prisoners — or, indeed, outside a context of presumptive entitlement to mental health care.

References

Adler, Freda. 1986. Jails as a repository for former mental patients. *International Journal of Offender Therapy & Comparative Criminology*, 30, 225–236.

American Bar Association. 1989. *ABA Criminal Justice Mental Health Standards*. Washington, DC: The Association.

American Psychiatric Association. 1974. *Clinical Aspects of the Violent Individual*. Washington, DC: The Association.

American Psychiatric Association. 1984. *Issues in Forensic Psychiatry*. Washington, DC: American Psychiatric Press.

American Psychiatric Association. 1987. *Diagnostic and Statistical Manual of Mental and Emotional Disorders, Third Edition, Revised*. Washington, DC: The Association.

Amnesty International. 1987. *United States of America: The Death Penalty*. London: Amnesty International.

Anastasi, Anne. 1988. *Psychological Testing*, 6th ed. New York: Macmillan.

Appelbaum, Paul S. 1988. The right to refuse treatment with antipsychotic medications: Retrospect and prospect. *American Journal of Psychiatry*, 145, 413–419.

Arboleda-Florez, Julio. 1981. Post-homicide psychotic reaction. *International Journal of Offender Therapy & Comparative Criminology*, 25, 47–52.

Atlas, Randy. 1984. Violence in prison: Environmental influences. *Environment & Behavior*, 16, 275–306.

Bailey, William C. 1976. Some further evidence on homicide and a regional culture of violence. *Omega: Journal of Death & Dying*, 7, 145–170.

Ball, John C., & David N. Nurco. 1984. Criminality during the life course of heroin addiction. *National Institute on Drug Abuse, Research Monograph Series, 49*. Pp. 305–312.

Ball, John C., Lawrence Rosen, John A. Flueck & David N. Nurco. 1982. Lifetime criminality of heroin addicts in the United States. *Journal of Drug Issues*, 12, 225–239.

Ball, John D., Robert P. Archer, Frederick A. Struve & John A. Hunter. 1987. MMPI correlates of a controversial EEG pattern among adolescent psychiatric patients. *Journal of Clinical Psychology*, 43, 708–714.

Baum, Maureen S., Ray E. Hosford & C. Scott Moss. 1984. Predicting violent behavior within a medium security correctional setting. *International Journal of Eclectic Psychotherapy*, 3, 18–24.

Beck, James C. & Edward A. Golowka. 1988. A study of enforced treatment in relation to Stone's "Thank You" theory. *Behavioral Sciences & the Law,* 6, 559–566.

Bell, Carl C. 1986. Coma and the etiology of violence. *Journal of the National Medical Association,* 78, 1167–1176.

Bell, Carl C. 1990. Neuropsychiatry and gun safety. *Journal of Neuropsychiatry & Clinical Neurosciences,* 2, 145–148.

Berkley, George E., Michael W. Giles, Jerry F. Hackett & Norman C. Kassoff. 1977. *Criminal Justice: Police, Courts, Corrections.* Boston: Holbrook.

Berkow, Robert J., & Andrew J. Fletcher. 1987. *The Merck Manual of Diagnosis and Therapy,* 15th ed. Rahway, NJ: Merck, Sharp & Dohme Research Laboratories.

Bernstein, Ira H., & Calvin P. Garbin. 1985. A simple set of salient weights for the major dimensions of MMPI scale variations. *Education & Psychological Measurement,* 45, 771–787.

Bernstein, Ira H., Gary Teng, Bruce D. Granneman & Calvin P. Garbin. 1987. Invariance in the MMPI's component structure. *Journal of Personality Assessment,* 51, 522–531.

Blackburn, Ronald. 1975-*a.* Aggression and the EEG: A quantitative analysis. *Journal of Abnormal Psychology,* 84, 359–365.

Blackburn, Ronald. 1975-*b.* An empirical classification of psychopathic personality. *British Journal of Psychiatry,* 127, 456–460.

Blackburn, Ronald. 1979. Cortical and autonomic arousal in primary and secondary psychopaths. *Psychophysiology,* 16, 143–150.

Block, Michael K., & William M. Rhodes. 1990. The impact of Federal sentencing guidelines. In Larry J. Siegel (ed.), *American Justice.* St. Paul, MN: West. Pp. 177–184.

Blum, Richard H. 1981. Violence, alcohol, and setting: An unexplored nexus. In James J. Collins, Jr. (ed.), *Drinking and Crime.* New York: Guilford. Pp. 110–142.

Blumstein, Alfred, & S. Moitra. 1981. Identification of "career criminals" from "chronic offenders" in a cohort. *Law & Policy Quarterly,* 2, 321–334.

Blumstein, Alfred, & Jacqueline Cohen. 1987. Characterizing criminal careers. *Science,* 237, 985–991.

Bohmer, Carol E. 1976. Bad or mad: The psychiatrist in the sentencing process. *Journal of Psychiatry & Law,* 4, 23–48.

Bohn, Martin J., & Gary S. Traub. 1986. Alienation of monolingual Hispanics in a Federal correctional institution. *Psychological Reports,* 59, 560–562.

Boulton, Alan A., Bruce A. Davis, Peter H. Yu, Stephen Wormith, & Donald Addington. 1983. Trace acid levels in the plasma and MAO activity in the platelets of violent offenders. *Psychiatry Research,* 8, 19–23.

Bradford, John M., & D. McLean. 1984. Sexual offenders, violence, and testosterone: A clinical study. *Canadian Journal of Psychiatry,* 29, 335–343.

Briar, Katharine H. 1983. Jails: Neglected asylums. *Social Casework,* 64, 1983, 387–393.

Brooks, Alexander D. 1986. The effect of law on the administration of antipsychotic medications. In Laurence Tancredi (ed.), *Ethical Issues in*

Epidemiologic Research. New Brunswick, NJ: Rutgers University Press. Pp. 183–200.

Brown, George W. 1986. Mental illness. In Linda H. Aiken & David Mechanic (eds.), *Applications of Social Science to Health Policy.* New Brunswick, NJ: Rutgers University Press. Pp. 175–203.

Brown, Phil, & Christopher J. Smith. 1988. Mental patients' rights: An empirical study of variation across the United States. *International Journal of Law & Psychiatry,* 11, 157–165.

Brown, Rosemary, Nigel Colter, Nicholas Corsellis, Timothy J. Crow, Christopher D. Frith, Roger Jagoe, Eve C. Johnstone & Laura Marsh. 1986. Postmortem evidence of structural brain changes in schizophrenia: Differences in brain weight, temporal horn area, and parahippocampal gyrus compared with affective disorder. *Archives of General Psychiatry,* 43, 36–42.

Bryant, Ernest T., Monte L. Scott, Christopher D. Tori, & Charles J. Golden. 1984. Neuropsychological deficits, learning disability, and violent behavior. *Journal of Consulting & Clinical Psychology,* 52, 323–324.

Budd, Robert D. 1982. The incidence of alcohol use in Los Angeles county homicide victims. *American Journal of Drug & Alcohol Abuse,* 9, 105–111.

Buikhuisen, Wouter. 1982. Aggressive behavior and cognitive disorders. *International Journal of Law & Psychiatry,* 5, 205–217.

Buikhuisen, Wouter, & B.W.G.P. Mejs. 1983. Psychosocial approach to recidivism. In Katherin [*sic*] T. van Dusen & Sarnoff A. Mednick (eds.), *Prospective Studies of Crime and Delinquency.* Boston: Kluwer-Nijhoff. Pp. 99–115.

Bukstel, Lee H., & Peter R. Kilmann. 1980. Psychological effects of imprisonment on confined individuals. *Psychological Bulletin,* 88, 469–493.

Bureau of the Census, U.S. Department of Commerce. 1988. *Profile of State Prison Inmates.* Washington, DC: Bureau of Justice Statistics, U.S. Department of Justice. Report NCJ- 109926.

Bureau of the Census, U.S. Department of Commerce. 1989. *Statistical Abstract of the United States.* Washington, DC: U.S. Government Printing Office.

Bureau of Justice Statistics. 1980. *Profile of Jail Inmates: National Prisoner Statistics Report* SD NPSJ-6, NCJ-65412. Washington, DC: U.S. Department of Justice.

Burke, Jack D., & Darrel A. Regier. 1988. Epidemiology of mental disorders. In John A. Talbott, Robert E. Hales & Stuart C. Yudofsky (eds.), *American Psychiatric Press Textbook of Psychiatry.* Washington, DC: American Psychiatric Press. Pp. 67–90.

Bush, John M. 1983. Criminality and psychopathology: Treatment for the guilty. *Federal Probation,* 47, 44–49.

Carbonell, Joyce L. 1983. Inmate classification: A cross-tabulation of two methods. *Criminal Justice & Behavior,* 10, 285–292.

Carbonell, Joyce L., Karen M. Moorhead & Edwin I. Megargee. 1984. Predicting prison adjustment with structured personality inventories. *Journal of Consulting & Clinical Psychology,* 52, 280–294.

Carlen, Pat. 1985. Law, psychiatry, and women's imprisonment: A sociological view. *British Journal of Psychiatry,* 146, 618–621.

Cavanaugh, James L., & Oriest E. Wasyliw. 1985. Treating the not guilty by reason of insanity outpatient: A two year study. *Bulletin of the American Academy of Psychiatry & the Law,* 13, 407–415.

Cicerone, Keith D., & Jeanne C. Wood. 1987. Planning disorder after closed head injury: A case study. *Archives of Physical Medicine & Rehabilitation,* 68, 111–115.

Clarke, Ronald V. 1980. "Situational" crime prevention. *British Journal of Criminology,* 20, 136–147.

Clarke, Ronald V. 1985. Delinquency, environment, and intervention. *Child Psychology & Psychiatry,* 26, 505–523.

Clarkin, John F., & Stephen W. Hurt. 1988. Psychological assessment: Tests and rating scales. In John A. Talbott, Robert E. Hales & Stuart C. Yudofsky (eds.), *American Psychiatric Press Textbook of Psychiatry.* Washington, DC: American Psychiatric Press. Pp. 225–246.

Cloninger, C. Robert, Theodore Reich & Samuel B. Guze. 1975. The multifactorial model of disease transmission: Sex differences in the familial transmission of sociopathy (antisocial personality). *British Journal of Psychiatry,* 127, 11–22.

Coccarro, Emil F., Larry J. Siever, Howard M. Klar & Gail Mauer. 1989. Serotonergic studies in patients with affective and personality disorders: Correlates with suicidal and impulsive aggressive behavior. *Archives of General Psychiatry,* 46, 587–599.

Cohen, Bruce M., Ferdinando Buonanno, Paul E. Keck, Seth P. Finkelstein, & Francine M. Benes. 1988. Comparison of MRI and CT scans in a group of psychiatric patients. *American Journal of Psychiatry,* 145, 1084–1088.

Colligan, Robert C., David Osborne, Wendell M. Swenson & Kenneth P. Offord. 1989. *The MMPI: A Contemporary Normative Study,* 2nd ed. Odessa, FL: Psychological Assessment Resources.

Collins, James J., Jr. 1981. Alcohol careers and criminal careers. In James J. Collins, Jr. (ed.), *Drinking and Crime.* New York: Guilford. Pp. 152–206.

Conacher, G. Neil. 1988. Pharmacotherapy of the aggressive adult patient. *International Journal of Law & Psychiatry,* 11, 205–212.

Cowen, Philip J. 1988. Prolactin response to tryptophan during mianserin treatment. *American Journal of Psychiatry,* 145, 740–741.

Cox, Verne C., Paul B. Paulus & Garvin McCain. 1984. Prison crowding research: The relevance for prison housing standards and a general approach regarding crowding phenomena. *American Psychologist,* 39, 1148–1160.

Coyle, Joseph T. 1988. Neuroscience and psychiatry. In John A. Talbott, Robert E. Hales & Stuart C. Yudofsky (eds.), *American Psychiatric Press Textbook of Psychiatry.* Washington, DC: American Psychiatric Press. Pp. 3–32.

Croughan, Jack L. 1985. The contribution of family studies to understanding drug abuse. In Lee N. Robins (ed.), *Studying Drug Abuse.* New Brunswick, NJ: Rutgers University Press. Pp. 93–116.

Cullen, Francis T., & Gilbert, Karen E. 1982. *Reaffirming Rehabilitation.* Cincinnati: Anderson.

Cullum, C. Munro, & Erin D. Bigler. 1988. Short form MMPI findings in patients with predominantly lateralized cerebral dysfunction: Neuropsychological and computerized axial tomography-derived parameters. *Journal of Nervous & Mental Disease,* 176, 332–342.

Dabbs, James M., Robert L. Frady, Timothy S. Carr, & Norma F. Besch. 1987. Saliva testosterone and criminal violence in young adult prison inmates. *Psychosomatic Medicine,* 49, 174–182.

Dahlstrom, W. Grant, James H. Panton, Kenneth P. Bain & Leona E. Dahlstrom. 1986. Utility of the Megargee & Bohn MMPI typological assessments: Study with a sample of death row inmates. *Criminal Justice & Behavior,* 13, 5–17.

Daniel, Anasseril E., Philip W. Harris & Sayed A. Husain. 1981. Differences between midlife female offenders and those younger than 40. *American Journal of Psychiatry,* 138, 1225–1228.

Daniel, Anasseril E., & Philip W. Harris. 1982. Female homicide offenders referred for pre-trial psychiatric examination: A descriptive study. *Bulletin of the American Academy of Psychiatry & the Law,* 10, 261–269.

Davis, Bruce A., et al. 1983. Correlative relationships between biochemical activity and aggressive behavior. *Progress in Nauro-psychopharmacology & Biological Psychiatry,* 7, 529–535.

Dawson, E.B, T.D. Moore & W.J. McGanity. 1972. Relationship of lithium metabolism to mental hospital admission and homicide. *Diseases of the Nervous System,* 33, 546–556.

Day, Lincoln H. 1984. Death from non-war violence: An international comparison. *Social Science & Medicine,* 19, 917–927.

Dembo, Richard, Mark Washburn, Eric D. Wish, James Schmeidler, Alan Getreu, Estellita Berry, Linda Williams & William R. Blount. 1987. Further examination of the association between marijuana use and crime among youths entering a juvenile detention center. *Journal of Psychoactive Drugs,* 19, 361–373.

Denkowski, George C., & Kathryn M. Denkowski. 1985. The mentally retarded offender in the state prison system: Identification, prevalence, adjustment, and rehabilitation. *Criminal Justice & Behavior,* 12, 55–70.

Denkowski, George C., & Kathryn M. Denkowski. 1986. Community-based residential treatment of the mentally retarded. *Journal of Community Psychology,* 13, *1985,* 299–305.

Denkowski, George C., Kathryn M. Denkowski, & Jerome Mabli. 1984. A residential treatment model for mentally retarded adolescent offenders. *Hospital & Community Psychiatry,* 35, 279–281.

Dix, George E. 1983. A legal perspective on dangerousness: Current status. *Psychiatric Annals,* 13, 243–256.

Doerner, William G. 1975. A regional analysis of homicide rates in the United States. *Criminology,* 13, 90–101.

Dwyer, Richard E. 1988. The employer's need to provide a safe working environment: Use and abuse of drug screening. *Labor Studies Journal,* 12, 3–19.

Edinger, Jack D. 1979. Cross-validation of the Megargee MMPl typology for prisoners. *Journal of Consulting & Clinical Psychology,* 47, 234–242.

Edinger, Jack D., David L. Reuterfors & S. Susan Logue, 1982. Cross-validation of the Megargee MMPI typology: A study of specialized inmate populations. *Criminal Justice & Behavior,* 9, 184–203.

Ekland-Olson, Sheldon. 1986. Crowding, social control, and prison violence: Evidence from the post-Ruiz years in Texas. *Law & Society Review*, 20, 389–421.

Erdman, Harold P., Marjorie H. Klein, John H. Greist & Sandra M. Bass. 1987. A comparison of the Diagnostic Interview Schedule and clinical diagnosis. *American Journal of Psychiatry*, 144, 1477–1480.

Feinberg, Stephen, & Gramsbach, Patricia. 1979. An assessment of the accuracy of "The effectiveness of correctional treatment." In Sechrest, Lee, Susan O. White & Elizabeth D. Brown. *The Rehabilitation of Criminal Offenders: Problems and Prospects*. Washington: National Academy of Sciences. Pp. 119–147.

Feldman, Robert S., & Linda F. Quenzer. 1984. *Fundamentals of Neuropsychopharmacology*. Sunderland, MA: Sinauer.

Felson, Richard B., & Henry J. Steadman. 1983. Situational factors in disputes leading to criminal violence. *Criminology*, 21, 59–74.

Felson, Richard B., & Henry J. Steadman. 1984. Self- reports of violence. *Criminology*, 22, 321–342.

Felson, Richard B., Stephen A. Ribner & Meryl S. Siegel. 1984. Age and the effect of third parties during criminal violence. *Sociology & Social Research*, 68, 452–462.

Fingarette, Herbert. 1988. *Heavy Drinking: The Myth of Alcoholism as a Disease*. Berkeley: University of California Press.

Fingarette, Herbert. 1990. We should reject the disease concept of alcoholism. *Harvard Medical School Mental Health Letter*, 6 (8), 4–6.

Finkle, Bryan S., & Kevin L. McCloskey. 1977. The forensic toxicology of cocaine. *National Institute on Drug Abuse Research Monograph Series 13: Cocaine*. Washington: NIDA.

Fishbain, David A., James R. Fletcher, Timothy E. Aldrich & Joseph H. Davis. 1987. Relationship between Russian roulette deaths and risk-taking behavior: A controlled study. *American Journal of Psychiatry*, 144, 563–567.

Flanagan, Timothy J., & Katherine M. Jamieson. 1988. *Sourcebook of Criminal Justice Statistics*. Washington, DC: Bureau of Justice Statistics, U.S. Department of Justice.

Fletcher, Jack M., Linda Ewing-Cobbs, Michael E. Miner, Harvey S. Levin & Howard M. Eisenberg. 1990. Behavioral changes after closed head injury in children. *Journal of Consulting & Clinical Psychology*, 58, 93–98.

Fowler, Raymond D. 1987. Assessment for decision in a correctional setting. In Donald R. Peterson & Daniel B. Fishman (eds.), *Assessment for Decision*. New Brunswick, NJ: Rutgers University Press. Pp. 214–239.

Fowles, George P. 1988. Neuropsychologically impaired offenders: Considerations for assessment and treatment. *Psychiatric Annals*, 18, 692–697.

Frances, Richard J., & John E. Franklin. 1987. Alcohol- induced organic mental disorders. In Robert E. Hales & Stuart C. Yudofsky (eds.), *American Psychiatric Press Textbook of Neuropsychiatry*. Washington, DC: American Psychiatric Press. Pp. 141–156.

Frances, Richard J., & John E. Franklin. 1988. Alcohol and other psychoactive substance abuse disorders. In John A. Talbott, Robert E. Hales & Stuart C. Yudofsky (eds.), *American Psychiatric Press Textbook of Psychiatry.* Washington, DC: American Psychiatric Press. Pp. 313–356.

Franzen, Michael D., & Mark R. Lovell. 1987. Neuropsychological assessment. In Robert E. Hales & Stuart C. Yudofsky (eds.), *American Psychiatric Press Textbook of Neuropsychiatry.* Washington, DC: American Psychiatric Press. Pp. 41–54.

Franzen, Michael D., & Carl Rollyn Sullivan. 1987. Cognitive rehabilitation of patients with neuropsychiatric disabilities. In Robert E. Hales & Stuart C. Yudofsky (eds.), *American Psychiatric Press Textbook of Neuropsychiatry.* Washington, DC: American Psychiatric Press. Pp. 439–450.

Frishtik, Mordechai. 1988. The probation officer's recommendations in his "investigation report." *Journal of Offender Rehabilitation,* 13, 101–132.

Fry, Lincoln J. 1985. Drug abuse and crime in a Swedish birth cohort. *British Journal of Criminology,* 25, 46–59.

Galski, Thomas, Kirtley E. Thornton, & David Shumsky. 1990. Brain dysfunction in sex offenders. *Journal of Offender Rehabilitation,* in press.

Garcia, Sandra A., & Robert Batey. 1988. Protecting forcibly institutionalized mental patients from unwanted drug therapy: A Fourth Amendment analysis, *Law & Psychology Review,* 12, 1–19.

Gastil, Raymond D. 1971. Homicide and a regional culture of violence. *American Sociological Review,* 36, 412–427.

Gearing, Milton L. 1979. The MMPI as a primary differentiator and predictor of behavior in prison: A methodological critique and review of the recent literature. *Psychological Bulletin,* 86, 929–963.

Gelberg, Lillian, Lawrence S. Linne & Barbara D. Leake. 1988. Mental health, alcohol and drug use, and criminal history among homeless adults. *American Journal of Psychiatry,* 145, 191–196.

Gendreau, Paul, & Ross, Bob. 1979. Effective correctional treatment: Bibliotherapy for cynics. *Crime & Delinquency,* 17, 463–489.

Gendreau, Paul, & Ross, Robert. 1981. Offender rehabilitation: The appeal of success. *Federal Probation,* 9, 45–47.

Gift, Thomas E., John S. Strauss, Barry A. Ritzler & Ronald F. Kokes. 1988. Social class and psychiatric disorder: The examination of an extreme. *Journal of Nervous & Mental Disease,* 176, 593–597.

Gilandas, Alex, Stephen Touyz, Pierre J.V. Beumont & H.P. Greenberg. 1984. *Handbook of Neuropsychological Assessment.* Sydney: Grune & Stratton.

Gillies, Hunter. 1976. Homicide in the west of Scotland. *British Journal of Psychiatry,* 128, 105–127.

Glaser, Daniel. 1976. Achieving better questions: A half century's progress in correctional research. *Federal Probation,* 4, 3–9.

Golann, Stuart, & William J. Fremouw (eds.). 1976. *The Right to Treatment for Mental Patients.* New York: Irvington.

Gordon, Alistair M. 1983. Drugs and delinquency: A ten- year follow-up of drug clinic patients. *British Journal of Psychiatry,* 142, 169–173.

Gorenstein, Ethan E. 1982. Frontal lobe functions in psychopaths. *Journal of Abnormal Psychology,* 91, 368–379.

Gorenstein, Ethan E., & Joseph P. Newman. 1980. Disinhibitory psychopathology: A new perspective and model for research. *Psychological Review,* 87, 301–315.

Gormally, J.G., Stanley L. Brodsky, C.B. Clements & Raymond D. Fowler. 1972. *Minimum Mental Health Standards for the Alabama Correctional System.* University, AL: Center for Correctional Psychology, University of Alabama.

Gove, Walter R. 1982. The labeling and treatment of mental illness in jails: A theoretical discussion. *Crime & Delinquency,* 82, 157–173.

Graham, John R. 1987. *The MMPI: A Practical Guide,* 2nd ed. New York: Oxford University Press.

Graham, Mary G. 1990. Controlling drug abuse and crime: A research update. In Larry J. Siegel (ed.), *American Justice.* St. Paul, MN: West. Pp. 101–113.

Greenberg, Stephanie W. 1981. Alcohol and crime: A methodological critique of the literature. In James J. Collins, Jr. (ed.), *Drinking and Crime.* New York: Guilford. Pp. 70–109.

Greene, Roger L. 1988. The relative efficacy of F-K and the obvious and subtle scales to detect overreporting of psychopathology on the MMPI. *Journal of Clinical Psychology,* 44, 152–159.

Gross, Lawrence S. 1987. Neuropsychiatric aspects of vitamin deficiency states. In Robert E. Hales & Stuart C. Yudofsky (eds.), *American Psychiatric Press Textbook of Neuropsychiatry.* Washington, DC: American Psychiatric Press. Pp. 287–306.

Gunn, John C. 1978. *Psychiatric Aspects of Imprisonment.* New York: Academic.

Gur, Raquel E., Susan M. Resnick, Ruben C. Gur, Abass Alavi, Stanley Caroff, Michael Kushner & Martin Reivich. 1987. Regional brain function in schizophrenia: Repeated evaluation with positron emission tomography. *Archives of General Psychiatry,* 44, 126–129.

Hall, Harold V. 1984. Predicting dangerousness for the courts. *American Journal of Forensic Psychology,* 2, 5–25.

Hall, Harold V., & Douglas McNinch. 1988. Linking crime-specific behavior to neuropsychological impairment. *International Journal of Clinical Neuropsychology,* 10, 113–122.

Halleck, Seymour L. 1987. *The Mentally Disordered Offender.* Washington, DC: American Psychiatric Press.

Hammersley, Richard, & Valerie Morrison. 1987. Effects of polydrug use on the criminal activities of heroin users. *British Journal of Addiction,* 82, 899–906

Hammersley, Richard, & Valerie Morrison. 1988. Crime amongst heroin, alcohol, and cannabis users. *Medicine & Law,* 7, 185–193.

Hare, Robert D. 1970. *Psychopathy: Theory and Research.* New York: John Wiley.

Hare, Robert D. 1979. Psychopathy and laterality of cerebral function. *Journal of Abnormal Psychology,* 88, 605–610.

Hare, Robert D. 1982. Psychopathy and physiological activity during anticipation of an aversive stimulus in a distraction paradigm. *Psychophysiology,* 19, 266–271.

Hare, Robert D. 1984. Performance of psychopaths on cognitive tasks related to frontal lobe function. *Journal of Abnormal Psychology,* 93, 133–140.

Hare, Robert D. 1985. Comparison of procedures for assessment of psychopathy. *Journal of Consulting & Clinical Psychology,* 53, 7–16.

Hare, Robert D., & Leslie M. McPherson. 1984. Psychopathy and perceptual asymmetry during verbal dichotic listening. *Journal of Abnormal Psychology,* 93, 141–149.

Hare, Robert D., & Leslie M. McPherson. 1985. Violent and aggressive behavior by criminal psychopaths. *International Journal of Law & Psychiatry,* 7, 35–50.

Hare, Robert D., Leslie M. McPherson & Adelle E. Forth. 1988. Male psychopaths and their criminal careers. *Journal of Consulting & Clinical Psychology,* 56, 710–714.

Hartman, David E. 1988. *Neuropsychological Toxicity.* New York: Pergamon.

Hathaway, Starke R., & Paul E. Meehl. 1956. Psychiatric implications of code types. In George S. Welsh & W. Grant Dahlstrom (eds.), *Basic Readings on the MMPI in Psychology and Medicine.* Minneapolis: University of Minnesota Press. Pp. 136–144.

Heather, Nick. 1976. Specificity of schizophrenic thought disorder: A replication and extension of previous findings. *British Journal of Social & Clinical Psychology,* 15, 131–137.

Heather, Nick. 1977. Personal illness in 'lifers' and the effects of longterm indeterminate sentences. *British Journal of Criminology,* 17, 378–386.

Heilbrun, Alfred B., & Mark R. Heilbrun. 1985. Psychopathy and dangerousness: Comparison, integration, and extension of two psychopathic typologies. *British Journal of Clinical Psychology,* 24, 181–195.

Heinrichs, Douglas W., & Robert W. Buchanan. 1988. Significance and meaning of neurological signs in schizophrenia. *American Journal of Psychiatry,* 145, 11–18.

Helgason, Tomas. 1986. Expectancy and outcome of mental disorders in Iceland. In Myrna M. Weissman, Jerome K. Myers & Catherine E. Ross (eds.), *Community Surveys of Psychiatric Disorders.* New Brunswick, NJ: Rutgers University Press. Pp. 221–238.

Henderson, Monika. 1983. An empirical classification of non-violent offenders using the MMPI. *Personality & Individual Difference,* 4, 671–677.

Herrnstein, Richard. 1990. Biology and crime. In Larry J. Siegel (ed.), *American Justice.* St. Paul, MN: West. Pp. 11–14.

Hirsch, Charles S., Norman B. Rushforth, Amasa B. Ford & Lester Adelson. 1973. Homicide and suicide in a metropolitan county: Longterm trends. *Journal of the American Medical Association,* 223, 900–905.

Hofmann, Frederick G., & Adele D. Hofmann. 1975. *A Handbook on Drug and Alcohol Abuse: The Biomedical Aspects.* New York: Oxford University Press.

Holcomb, William R., & Nicholas A. Adams. 1985. Personality mechanisms of alcohol-related violence. *Journal of Clinical Psychology,* 41, 714–722.

Holland, Terrill R., & Bill McGarvey. 1985. Crime specialization, seriousness progression, and Markov chains. *Journal of Consulting & Clinical Psychology,* 52, 837–840.

Holland, Terril R., Gerald B. Beckett, & Norman Holt. 1982. Prediction of violent versus nonviolent recidivism from prior violent and non-violent criminality. *Journal of Abnormal Psychology*, 91, 178–182.

Holland, Terrill R., Gerald E. Beckett & Mario Levi. 1981. Intelligence, personality, and criminal violence: A multivariate analysis. *Journal of Consulting & Clinical Psychology*, 49, 106–111.

Hollin, Clive R. 1990. Cognitive-Behavioral Interventions with Young Offenders. New York: Pergamon.

Hollinger, Paul C. 1979. Violent deaths among the young: Recent trends in suicide, homicide, and accidents. *American Journal of Psychiatry*, 136, 1144–1147.

Hollinger, Paul C. 1980. Violent deaths as a leading cause of mortality: An epidemiologic study of suicide, homicide, and accidents. *American Journal of Psychiatry*, 137, 472–476.

Hollinger, Paul C., & Elaine H. Klemen. 1982. Violent deaths in the United States, 1900–1975: Relationships between suicide, homicide, and accidental deaths. *Social Science & Medicine*, 16, 1928–1938.

Hollingshead, August B., & Frederick C. Redlich. 1958. *Social Class and Mental Illness*. New York: John Wiley.

Hollingshead, August B. 1986. Social class and mental illness. In Myrna M. Weissman, Jerome K. Myers & Catherine E. Ross (eds.), *Community Surveys of Psychiatric Disorders*. New Brunswick, NJ: Rutgers University Press. Pp. 109–132.

Howard, Richard C. 1984. The clinical EEG and personality in mentally abnormal offenders. *Psychological Medicine*, 14, 569–580.

Hucker, S., R. Langevin, G. Wortzman, & J. Bain. 1986. Neuropsychological impairment in pedophiles. *Canadian Journal of Behavioural Science*, 18, 440–448.

Humphrey, John A., & Harriet J. Kupferer. 1977. Pockets of violence: An exploration of homicide and suicide. *Diseases of the Nervous System*, 38, 833–837.

Hunt, Dana E., Douglas S. Lipton & Barry Spunt. 1984. Patterns of criminal activity among methadone clients and current narcotics users not in treatment. *Journal of Drug Issues*, 14, 687–702.

Ilfeld, Frederic W., Jr. 1978. Psychological status of community residents along major demographic dimensions. *Archives of General Psychiatry*, 35, 716–724.

Inciardi, James A. 1982. The production and detection of fraud in street studies of crime and drugs. *Journal of Drug Issues*, 12, 285–291.

Inciardi, James A., Anne E. Pottieger & Charles E. Faupel. 1982. Black women, heroin, and crime: Some empirical notes. *Journal of Drug Issues*, 12, 241–250.

Jackson, George W. 1986. Substance abuse: Special issue. *Seminars in Occupational Medicine*, 1, 4 (Entire issue).

Johnson, Dennis L., James G. Simmons & B. Carl Gordon. 1983. Temporal consistency of the Meyer-Megargee inmate typology. *Criminal Justice & Behavior*, 10, 263–268.

Johnson, (Hon.) Frank M. 1976. Minimum constitutional standards for inmates of Alabama penal system. Appendix A, *Pugh v. Locke. 406 Federal Supplement,* 1976, 332–337.

Joint Commission on Accreditation of Hospitals. 1983. *Consolidated Standards Manual for Child, Adolescent, and Adult Psychiatric, Alcoholism, and Drug Abuse Facilities.* Chicago: The Commission.

Jones, Taz, William B. Beidelman & Raymond O. Fowler. 1981. Differentiating violent and non-violent prison inmates by use of selected MMPI scales. *Journal of Clinical Psychology,* 37, 673–678.

Joseph, Rhawn. 1990. *Neuropsychology, Neuropsychiatry, and Behavioral Neurology.* New York: Plenum.

Jutai, Jeffrey W., Robert D. Hare & John F. Connolly. 1987. Psychopathy and event-related brain potentials (ERPs) associated with attention to speech stimuli. *Personality & Individual Differences,* 8, 175–184.

Kaplan, Edith. 1990. The process approach to neuropsychological assessment of psychiatric patients. *Journal of Neuropsychiatry & Clinical Neurosciences,* 2, 72–87.

Keltikangas-Jarvinen, Liisa [*sic*]. 1978. Personality of violent offenders and suicidal individuals. *Psychiatrica Fennica,* 14, 57–63.

Kennedy, Thomas D. 1986. Trends in inmate classification: A status report of two computerized psychometric approaches. *Criminal Justice & Behavior,* 13, 165–184.

Klein, Stephen, Joan Petersilia & Susan Turner. 1990. Race and imprisonment decisions in California. *Science,* 247, 812–816.

Kolb, Douglas, & E.K. Eric Gunderson. 1985. Research on alcohol abuse and rehabilitation in the U.S. Navy. In Marc A. Schuckit (ed.), *Alcohol Patterns & Problems.* New Brunswick, NJ: Rutgers University Press. Pp. 157–178.

Krakowski, Menahem I., Antonio Convit, Judith Jaeger & Shang Lin. 1989. Neurological impairment in violent schizophrenic inpatients. *American Journal of Psychiatry,* 146, 849–853.

Kramer, Morton. 1977. *Psychiatric Services and the Changing Institutional Scene, 1950–1985.* Washington: U.S. Government Printing Office.

Kruesi, Markus J., Judith L. Rapoport, E. Mark Cummings & Carol J. Berg. 1987. Effects of sugar and aspartame on aggression and activity in children. *American Journal of Psychiatry,* 144, 1487–1490.

Kunce, Joseph T., Joseph J. Ryan & C. Cleary Eckelman. 1976. Violent behavior and differential WAIS characteristics. *Journal of Consulting & Clinical Psychology,* 44, 42–45.

Lamb, H. Richard. 1988. Community psychiatry and prevention. In John A. Talbott, Robert E. Hales & Stuart C. Yudofsky (eds.), *American Psychiatric Press Textbook of Psychiatry.* Washington, DC: American Psychiatric Press. Pp. 1141–1160.

Lamb, H. Richard, & Robert W. Grant. 1982. The mentally ill in an urban county jail. *Archives of General Psychiatry,* 39, 17–22.

Landesman, Sharon, & Earl C. Butterfield. 1987. Normalization and deinstitutionalization of mentally retarded individuals: Controversy and facts. *American Psychologist,* 42, 809–816.

Langevin, Ron, Mark Ben-Aron, George Wortzman, & Robert Dickey. 1987. Brain damage, diagnosis, and substance abuse among violent offenders. *Behavioral Sciences & the Law*, 5, 77–94.

Langevin, R., D. Paitich, B. Orchard, L. Handy & A. Russon. 1982-*a*. Diagnosis of killers seen for psychiatric assessment. *Acta Psychiatrica Scandinavica*, 66, 216–228.

Langevin, R., D. Paitich, B. Orchard, L. Handy & A. Russon. 1982-*b*. The role of alcohol, drugs, suicide attempts and situational strains in homicide committed by offenders seen for psychiatric assessment. *Acta Psychiatrica Scandinavica*, 66, 229–242.

Leighton, Dorothea C., Alexander H. Leighton, & R.A. Armstrong. 1968. Community psychiatry in a rural area: A social psychiatric approach. In Leopold Bellak (ed.), *Handbook of Community Psychiatry*. New York: Grune & Stratton.

Lemkau, Paul V. 1961. Notes on the development of mental hygiene in the Johns Hopkins School of Hygiene and Public Health. *Bulletin of the History of Medicine*, 35, 169–174.

Lemkau, Paul V. 1986. The 1933 and 1936 studies on the prevalence of mental illnesses in the Eastern Health District of Baltimore, Maryland. In Myrna M. Weissman, Jerome K. Myers & Catherine E. Ross (eds.), *Community Surveys of Psychiatric Disorders*. New Brunswick, NJ: Rutgers University Press. Pp. 23–40.

Leong, Gregory B. 1987. Outpatient civil commitment. *American Journal of Psychiatry*, 144, 694–695.

Levenson, Hanna. 1974. Multidimensional locus of control in prison inmates. *Personality & Social Psychology Bulletin*, 1, 354–356.

Levin, Jerome D. 1987. *Treatment of Alcoholism and Other Addictions*. Northvale, NJ: Jason Aronson.

Lewis, Collins E., C. Robert Cloninger & John Pais. 1983. Alcoholism, antisocial personality, and drug use in a criminal population. *Alcohol and Alcoholism*, 18, 53–60.

Lidberg, Lars. 1985. Platelet monoamine oxidase activity and psychopathy. *Psychiatry Research*, 16, 339–343.

Lindgren, Scott D., Dennis C. Harper, Lynn C. Richman & James A. Stebbens. 1986. Mental imbalance and the prediction of recurrent delinquent behavior. *Journal of Clinical Psychology*, 42, 821–825.

Lipton, Douglas, Robert Martinson & Judith Wilks. 1975. *The Effectiveness of Correctional Treatment: A Survey of Treatment Evaluation Studies*. New York: Praeger.

Litwack, Thomas R., & Louis B. Schlesinger. 1987. Assessing and predicting violence: Research, law, and applications. In Irving B. Weiner & Allen K. Hess (eds.), *Handbook of Forensic Psychology*. New York: Wiley. Pp. 205–257.

Loeber, Rolf. 1982. The stability of antisocial and delinquent child behavior: A review. *Child Development*, 53, 1431–1446.

Louscher, P. Kent, Ray E. Hosford & C. Scott Moss. 1983. Predicting dangerous behavior in a penitentiary using the Megargee typology. *Criminal Justice & Behavior*, 10, 269–284.

Luckenbill, David F. 1977. Criminal homicide as a situated transaction. *Social Problems*, 25, 175–186.

Luxenbrg, Jay S., Susan E. Swedo, Martine F. Flament, Robert P. Friedland, Judith Rapoport, & Stanley L. Rapoport. 1988. Neuroanatomical abnormalities in obsessive compulsive disorder detected with quantitative X-ray computed tomography. *American Journal of Psychiatry*, 145, 1089–1093.

Mabli, Jerome. 1985. Pre-release stress in prison inmates. *Journal of Offender Rehabilitation*, 8, 43–56.

MacKenzie, Doris L., & Lynne Goodstein. 1985. Long-term incarceration impacts and characteristics of long-term offenders: An empirical analysis. *Criminal Justice & Behavior*, 12, 395–414.

Maloney, Michael P., & Michael P. Ward. 1979. *Psychological Assessment: A Conceptual Approach*. New York: Oxford University Press.

Manderscheid, Ronald W., Michael J. Witkin, Marilyn J. Rosenstein, Laura J. Milazzo-Sayre, Helen E. Bethel & Robin L. MacAskill. 1985. Specialty mental health services: System and patient characteristics. In Carl A. Taube & Sally A. Barrett (eds.), *Mental Health, United States 1985*. Rockville, MD: Division of Biometry & Epidemiology, National Institute of Mental Health, U.S. Department of Health & Human Services. Pp. 7–69.

Martin, Martha B., Cynthia M. Owen & John M. Morisha. 1987. An overview of neurotransmitter and neuroreceptors. In Robert E. Hales & Stuart C. Yudofsky (eds.), *American Psychiatric Press Textbook of Neuropsychiatry*. Washington, DC: American Psychiatric Press. Pp. 55–87.

Martin, Ronald L., C. Robert Cloninger & Samuel B. Guze. 1982. The natural history of somatization and substance abuse in women criminals: A six year follow-up. *Comprehensive Psychiatry*, 23, 528–537.

Martinius, Joest. 1983. Homicide of an aggressive adolescent boy with right temporal lesion. *Neuroscience & BioBehavioral Reviews*, 7, 419–422.

Martinson, Robert. 1974. What works? — Questions and answers about prison reform. *The Public Interest*, 35, 22–54.

Martinson, Robert. 1976. California research at the crossroads. *Crime & Delinquency*, 14, 189–199.

Mawson, A.R., & Keith W. Jacobs. 1978. Corn consumption, tryptophan, and cross-national homicide rates. *Journal of Orthomolecular Psychiatry*, 7, 227–230.

Mayer, Connie. 1990. *Survey of Case Law Establishing Constitutional Minima for the Provision of Mental Health Services to Psychiatrically Involved Inmates*. Albany, NY: Albany Law School.

McAfee, James K., & Michele Gural. 1988. Individuals with mental retardation and the criminal justice system: The view from states' attorneys. *Mental Retardation*, 26, 5–12.

McClain, Paula D. 1982. Black female homicide offenders and victims: Are they from the same population? *Death Education*, 6, 265–278.

McCreary, Charles P. 1976. Trait and type differences among male and female assaultive and non-assaultive offenders. *Journal of Personality Assessment*, 40, 617–621.

McGarrell, Edmund F., & Timothy J. Flanagan. 1985. *Sourcebook of Criminal Justice Statistics*. Washington, DC: Bureau of Justice Statistics, U.S. Department of Justice.

McGlothlin, William H. 1985. Distinguishing effects from concomitants of drug use: The case of crime. In Lee N. Robins (ed.), *Studying Drug Abuse: Series in Psychosocial Epidemiology, VI*. New Brunswick, NJ: Rutgers University Press. Pp. 153–172.

McGovern, Francis J., & Jeffrey S. Nevid. 1986. Evaluation apprehension on psychological inventories in a prison-based setting. *Journal of Consulting & Clinical Psychology*, 54, 576–578.

McKinley, J. Charnley, & Starke R. Hathaway. 1956. Scales 3 (Hysteria), 9 (Hypomania), and 4 (Psychopathic deviate). In George S. Welsh & W. Grant Dahlstrom (eds.), *Basic Readings on the MMPI in Psychology and Medicine*. Minneapolis: University of Minnesota Press. Pp. 87–103.

McManus, Michael, Norman E. Alessi, W. Lexington Grapentine & Arthur S. Brickman. 1984. Psychiatric disturbances in serious delinquents. *Journal of the American Academy of Child Psychiatry*, 23, 602–615.

Mechanic, David. 1980. *Mental Health and Social Policy*, 2d ed. Englewood Cliffs: Prentice Hall.

Megargee, Edwin I. 1966. Undercontrolled and overcontrolled personality types in extreme antisocial aggression. *Psychological Monographs*, 80, 3 (Number 611).

Megargee, Edwin I., 1977. New classification system for criminal offenders. *Criminal Justice & Behavior*, 4, 1–116.

Megargee, Edwin I. 1986. A psychometric study of incarcerated presidential threateners. *Criminal Justice & Behavior*, 13, 243–260.

Megargee, Edwin I., & Martin J. Bohn. 1977. Empirically-determined characteristics of the ten types. *Criminal Justice & Behavior*, 4, 149–210.

Megargee, Edwin I., & Joyce L. Carbonell. 1985. Predicting prison adjustment with MMPI correctional scales. *Journal of Consulting & Clinical Psychology*, 53, 874–883.

Megargee, Edwin I., & Patrick E. Cook. 1975. Negative response bias and the MMPI overcontrolled hostility scale. *Journal of Consulting & Clinical Psychology*, 43, 725–729.

Megargee, Edwin I., J.C. Cook & H.T. Mendelsohn. 1967. The development and validation of an MMPI scale of assaultiveness in over-controlled individuals. *Journal of Abnormal Psychology*, 72, 519–528.

Megargee, Edwin I., Martin J. Bohn, James Meyer & Frances Sink. 1979. *Classifying Criminal Offenders: A New System Based on the MMPI*. Beverly Hills: Sage.

Meloy, J. Reid. 1988. *The Psychopathic Mind: Origins, Dynamics, Treatment*. Northvale, NJ: Jason Aronson.

Messner, Steven F. 1982. Poverty, inequality, and the urban homicide rate: Some unexpected findings. *Criminology*, 20, 103–114.

Messner, Steven F. 1983. Regional and racial effect on the urban homicide rate: The subculture of violence revisited. *American Journal of Sociology*, 88, 997–1007.

Messner, Steven F. 1985. Regional differences in the economic correlates of urban homicide rate: Some evidence on the importance of cultural context. *Criminology*, 21, 477–488.

Miller, Harry L. 1977. The "right to treatment": Can the courts rehabilitate and cure? The *Public Interest*, 46, 96–118.

Miller, S.J., Simon Dinitz & J. P. Conrad. 1982. *Careers of the Violent.* Lexington, MA: Heath.

Monahan, John. 1981-a. *The Clinical Prediction of Violent Behavior.* Washington, DC: U.S. Department of Health & Human Services.

Monahan, John. 1981-b. *Predicting Violent Behavior: An Assessment of Clinical Techniques.* Beverly Hills: Sage.

Monahan, John, & Henry J. Steadman. 1982. Crime and mental disorder: An epidemiological approach. In Michael Tonry & Norval Morris (eds.), *Crime and Justice,* IV. Chicago: University of Chicago Press.

Morand, Claud, Simon M. Young & Frank R. Ervin. 1983. Clinical response of aggressive schizophrenics to oral tryptophan. *Biological Psychiatry,* 18, 575–578.

Morris, Norval. 1974. *The Future of Imprisonment.* Chicago: University of Chicago Press.

Morris, Norval, & Michael Tonry. 1990. Between prison and probation — Intermediate punishments in a rational sentencing system. *Correctional Psychologist,* 22 (2), 1–7.

Morrissey, Elizabeth R. 1985. Methodologic issues in the study of special populations. In Marc A. Schuckit (ed.), *Alcohol Patterns and Problems.* New Brunswick, NJ: Rutgers University Press. Pp. 79–111.

Moss, C. Scott, Mark E. Johnson & Ray E. Hosford. 1984. An assessment of the Megargee typology in lifelong criminal violence. *Criminal Justice & Behavior,* 11, 225–234.

Motiuk, Laurence L., James Bonta & Don A. Andrews. 1986. Classification in halfway houses: The relative and incremental predictive criterion validities of the Megargee MMPI and LSI systems. *Criminal Justice & Behavior,* 13, 33–46.

Mrad, David F., Robert I. Kabacoff & Paul Duckro. 1983. Validation of the Megargee typology in a halfway house setting. *Criminal Justice & Behavior,* 10, 252–262.

Murphy, Jane M. 1986. The Stirling County study. In Myrna M. Weissman, Jerome K. Myers & Catherine E. Ross (eds.), *Community Surveys of Psychiatric Disorders.* New Brunswick, NJ: Rutgers University Press. Pp. 133–154.

Myers, Jerome K., & Myrna M. Weissman. 1986. Psychiatric disorders in a U.S. urban community: The New Haven study. In Myrna M. Weissman, Jerome K. Myers & Catherine E. Ross (eds.), *Community Surveys of Psychiatric Disorders.* New Brunswick, NJ: Rutgers University Press. Pp. 155–176.

Nathan, Peter E., & Anne-Helene Skinstad. 1987. Outcomes of treatment for alcohol problems: Current methods, problems, and results. *Journal of Consulting & Clinical Psychology,* 55, 332–340.

National Center for State Courts, U.S. Department of Justice. 1979. *State Court Caseload Statistics.* Washington, DC: National Criminal Justice Statistics and Information Service.

Nemeroff, Charles B., Michael J. Owens, Garth Bissette, Anne C. Andorn & Michael Stanley. 1988. Reduced corticotropin releasing factor binding sites in the frontal cortex of suicide victims. 1988. *Archives of General Psychiatry,* 45, 577–579.

Newcomb, Michael D., & P.M. Bentler. 1988. Impact of adolescent drug use and social support on problems of young adults: A longitudinal study. *Journal of Abnormal Psychology,* 97, 64–75.

Nurco, David N., John C. Ball, John W. Shaffer & Thomas E. Hanlon. 1985. The criminality of narcotic addicts. *Journal of Nervous & Mental Disease,* 173, 94–102.

Nurco, David N., John W. Shaffer, John C. Ball & Timothy W. Kinlock. 1984. Trends in the commission of crime among narcotic addicts over successive periods of addiction and nonaddiction. *American Journal of Drug & Alcohol Abuse,* 10, 481–489.

O'Brien, Robert M. 1987. The interracial nature of violent crimes: A re-examination. *American Journal of Sociology,* 92, 817–835.

Ojesjo, Leif. 1983. Alcohol, drugs, and forensic psychiatry. *Psychiatric Clinics of North America,* 6, 733–749.

Olfson, Mark. 1987. Weir Mitchell and lithium bromide. *American Journal of Psychiatry,* 144, 1101–1102.

Orvaschel, Helen, Diane Sholomskas & Myrna Weissman. 1980. Assessing children in psychiatric epidemiological studies: A review of interview techniques. In Felton Earls (ed.), *Studies of Children: Psychosocial Epidemiology.* New York: Prodist/Neal Watson. Pp. 84–95.

Pallone, Nathaniel J. 1986. *On the Social Utility of Psychopathology: A Deviant Majority and Its Keepers?* New Brunswick, NJ: Transaction Books.

Pallone, Nathaniel J. 1989. Controlled dangerous substances and felony crime: Data from recent studies in the US. In Raagnar Waahlberg (ed.), *Prevention and Control: Realities and Aspirations,* Volume III. Oslo: National Directorate for the Prevention of Alcohol & Drug Problems. Pp. 498–507.

Pallone, Nathaniel J. 1990-*a.* Drug use and felony crime: Biochemical credibility and unsettled questions. *Journal of Offender Rehabilitation,* 15, 85–109.

Pallone, Nathaniel J. 1990-*b. Rehabilitating Criminal Sexual Psychopaths: Legislative Mandates, Clinical Quandaries.* New Brunswick, NJ: Transaction Books.

Pallone, Nathaniel J., & James J. Hennessy. 1977. Some correlates of recidivism among misdemeanants and minor felons. *Journal of Social Psychology,* 101, 321–322.

Pallone, Nathaniel J., & Richard J. Tirman. 1978. Correlates of substance abuse remission in alcoholism rehabilitation: Effective treatment or symptom abandonment? *Journal of Offender Rehabilitation,* 3, 7–18.

Pallone, Nathaniel J., & Daniel S. LaRosa. 1979. Mental health specialists and services in correctional facilities: Who does what? *Journal of Offender Rehabilitation,* 4, 33–41.

Pallone, Nathaniel J., James J. Hennessy & Daniel S. LaRosa. 1980. Professional psychology in state correctional institutions: Present status and alternate futures. *Professional Psychology,* 11, 755–763.

Panton, James H. 1977. Personality characteristics of drug pushers incarcerated within a state prison population. *Quarterly Journal of Corrections,* 1, 11–13.

Panton, James H. 1978. Personality differences between rapists of adults, rapists of children, and non-violent sexual molesters of female children. *Research Communications in Psychology, Psychiatry & Behavior,* 3, 385–393.

Panton, James H. 1979. MMPI profile configurations associated with incestuous and non-incestuous child molesting. *Psychological Reports,* 45, 335–338.

Parisi, Nicolette, Michael R. Gottfredson, Michael J. Hindelang, & Timothy J. Flanagan. 1979. *Sourcebook of Criminal Justice Statistics.* Washington, DC: Bureau of Justice Statistics, U.S. Department of Justice.

Pasamanick, Benjamin. 1962. A survey of mental disease in an urban population. *American Journal of Psychiatry,* 119, 299 305.

Penrose, Lionel S. 1939. Mental disease and crime: Outline of a comparative study of European statistics. *Mcdical Psychology,* 19, 1–15.

Pernanen, Kai. 1981. Theoretical aspects of the relationship between alcohol use and crime. In James J. Collins, Jr. (ed.), *Drinking and Crime.* New York: Guilford. Pp. 1–69.

Perry, Samuel. 1987. Substance-induced organic mental disorders. In Robert E. Hales & Stuart C. Yudofsky (eds.), *American Psychiatric Press Textbook of Neuropsychiatry.* Washington, DC: American Psychiatric Press. Pp. 157–176.

Petersen, K.G. Ingemar, M. Matousek, Sarnoff A. Mednick, J. Volavka & V. Pollock. 1982. EEG antecedents of thievery. *Acta Psychiatrica Scandinavica,* 65, 331–338.

Petersilia, Joan. 1980. Criminal career research: A review of recent evidence. In Norval Morris & Michael Tonry (eds.), *Crime and Justice, II.* Chicago: University of Chicago Press. Pp. 321–379.

Peterson, Donald R. 1987. The role of assessment in professional psychology. In Donald R. Peterson & Daniel B. Fishman (eds.), *Assessment for Decision.* New Brunswick, NJ: Rutgers University Press. Pp. 5–43.

Peterson, Ruth D., & John Hagan. 1984. Changing conceptions of race: Towards an account of anomalous findings of sentencing research. *American Sociological Review,* 49, 56–70.

Petursson, Hannes, & Gisli H. Gundjonsson. 1981. Psychiatric aspects of homicide. *Acta Psychiatrica Scandinavica,* 64, 363–371.

Phillips, Michael R., Aron S. Wolf & David J. Coons. 1988. Psychiatry and the criminal justice system: Testing the myths. *American Journal of Psychiatry,* 145, 605–610.

Pichot, Pierre. 1978. Psychopathic behaviour: A historical overview. In Robert D. Hare & Daisy Schalling (eds.), *Psychopathic Behaviour: Approaches to Research.* New York: John Wiley. Pp. 56–70.

Pilchard, D.A. 1979. Stable predictors of recidivism: A summary. *Criminology,* 17, 15–21.

Polich, J. Michael, & Charles T. Kaelber. 1985. Sample surveys and the epidemiology of alcoholism. In Marc A. Schuckit (ed.), *Alcohol Patterns and Problems.* New Brunswick, NJ: Rutgers University Press. Pp. 43–77.

President's Commission on Law Enforcement and Administration of Justice. 1967. *Task Force Report: Science and Technology.* Washington, DC: U.S. Government Printing Office.

Pruesse, M., & Vernon L. Quinsey. 1977. Dangerousness of patients released from maximum security—A replication. *Journal of Psychiatry & Law,* 5, 217–224.

Pruitt, Charles R., & James Q. Wilson. 1983. A longitudinal study of the effect of race on sentencing. *Law & Society Review,* 17, 613–635.

Rada, Richard, D.R. Laws, Robert Kellner, Laxmi Stivasta, & Glenn Peake. 1983. Plasma androgens in violent and non-violent sex offenders. *Bulletin of the American Academy of Psychiatry & the Law,* 11, 149–158.

Radloff, Lenore Sawyer, & Ben Z. Locke. 1986. The community mental health assessment survey and the CES-D scale. In Myrna M. Weissman, Jerome K. Myers & Catherine E. Ross (eds.), *Community Surveys of Psychiatric Disorders.* New Brunswick, NJ: Rutgers University Press. Pp. 177–190.

Raine, Adrian, & Peter H. Venables. 1988. Enhanced P3 evoked potentials and longer P3 recovery times in psychopaths. *Psychophysiology,* 25, 30–38.

Robins, Lee N. 1985. Epidemiology: Reflections on testing the validity of psychiatric interviews. *Archives of General Psychiatry,* 42, 918–824.

Rodenhauser, Paul. 1984. Treatment refusal in a forensic hospital: Ill use of the lasting right. *Bulletin of the American Academy of Psychiatry & the Law,* 12, 59–63.

Rodenhauser, Paul, Charles E. Schwenkner & H.J. Khamis. 1987. Factors related to drug treatment refusal in a forensic hospital. *Hospital & Community Psychiatry,* 38, 631–637.

Rogers, Richard. 1986. *Conducting Insanity Evaluations.* New York: Van Nostrand Reinhold.

Rogers, Richard. 1987. APA's position on the insanity defense: Empiricism versus emotionalism. *American Psychologist,* 42, 840–848.

Rohrbeck, Cynthia A., & Craig T. Twentyman. 1986. Multimodal assessment of impulsiveness in abusing, neglecting, and nonmaltreating mothers and their preschool children. *Journal of Consulting & Clinical Psychology,* 54, 231–236.

Roizen, Judy. 1981. Alcohol and criminal behavior among blacks: The case for research on special populations. In James J. Collins, Jr. (ed.), *Drinking and Crime.* New York: Guilford. Pp. 207–252.

Rosen, Lee A., Sharon R. Booth, Mary E. Pender, Melanie L. McGrath, Sue Sorrell & Ronald S. Drabman. 1988. Effects of sugar (sucrose) on children's behavior. *Journal of Consulting & Clinical Psychology,* 56, 583–589.

Rosenthal, Barry J., & Kareem Nakkash. 1982. Drug addiction and criminality: A model for predicting the incidence of crime among a treatment population. *Journal of Drug Issues,* 12, 293–303.

Rosse, Richard B., & John M. Morisha. 1988. Laboratory and other diagnostic tests in psychiatry. In John A. Talbott, Robert E. Hales & Stuart C. Yudofsky (eds.), *American Psychiatric Press Texbook of Psychiatry.* Washington, DC: American Psychiatric Press. Pp. 247–277.

Rosse, Richard B., Cynthia M. Owen & John M. Morisha. 1987. Brain imaging and laboratory testing in neuropsychiatry. In Robert E. Hales & Stuart C. Yudofsky (eds.), *American Psychiatric Press Textbook of Neuropsychiatry.* Washington, DC: American Psychiatric Press. Pp. 17–40.

Roundtree, George A., Dan W. Edwards & Jack B. Parker. 1984. A study of the personal characteristics of probationers as related to recidivism. *Journal of Offender Rehabilitation,* 8, 53–61.

Ruback, R. Barry, & Timothy S. Carr. 1984. Crowding in a woman's prison: Attitudinal and behavioral effects. *Journal of Applied Social Psychology,* 14, 57–68.

Rubinson, Eileen, Gregory M. Asnis & Jill H. Friedman. 1988. Knowledge of the diagnostic criteria for major depression: A survey of mental health professionals. *Journal of Nervous & Mental Disease,* 176, 480–484.

Ruff, Carol F., Joyce L. Ayers & Donald I. Templer. 1977. The Watson and the Hovey MMPI scales: Do they measure organicity or functional psychopathology? *Journal of Clinical Psychology,* 33, 732–734.

Sandhu, Harjit S. 1977. *Modern Corrections: The Offenders, Therapies, and Community Integration.* Springfield, IL: Charles C. Thomas.

Schatzberg, Alan F., & Jonathan O. Cole. 1986. *Manual of Clinical Psychopharmacology.* Washington: American Psychiatric Press.

Schoenthaler, Stephen J. 1982. The effect of sugar on the treatment and control of antisocial behavior: A double-blind study of an incarcerated juvenile population. *International Journal of Biosocial Research,* 3, 1–9.

Schoenthaler, Stephen J. 1983-*a*. Diet and crime: An empirical examination of the value of nutrition in the control and treatment of incarcerated juvenile offenders. *International Journal of Biosocial Research,* 4, 23–59.

Schoenthaler, Stephen J. 1983-*b*. The Los Angeles probation department diet-behavior program: An empirical analysis of six institutional settings. *International Journal of Biosocial Research,* 5, 88–98.

Schoenthaler, Stephen J. 1983-*c*. The northern California diet-behavior program: An empirical examination of 3000 incarcerated juveniles in Stanislaus County juvenile hall. *International Journal of Biosocial Research,* 5, 99–106.

Schoentaler, Stephen J. 1983-*d*. Types of offenses which can be reduced in an institutional setting using nutritional intervention. *International Journal of Biosocial Research,* 4, 74–84.

Schofield, William. 1986. *Psychotherapy: The Purchase of Friendship,* 2nd ed. New Brunswick, NJ: Transaction.

Schneider, A.L., P.R. Schneider & S.G. Bazemore. 1981. In-program reoffense rates for juveniles in restitution projects. In *Oversight Hearing on Juvenile Restitution Programs,* NIJ Document 82247. Rockville, MD: National Institute for Juvenile Justice & Delinquency Prevention, U.S. Department of Justice. Pp. 286–368.

Schuckit, Marc A., Gerard Herrman & Judith J. Schuckit. 1977. The importance of psychiatric illness in newly arrested prisoners. *Journal of Nervous & Mental Disease,* 165, 118–125.

Scull, Andrew. 1984. *Decarceration: Community Treatment and the Deviant, A Radical View*, New Brunswick, NJ: Rutgers University Press.

Sechrest, Lee, Susan O. White & Elizabeth D. Brown. 1979. *The Rehabilitation of Criminal Offenders: Problems and Prospects.* Washington: National Academy of Sciences.

Shah, Saleem A. 1976. Community mental health and the criminal justice system: Some issues and problems. In John Monahan (ed.), *Community Mental Health and the Criminal Justice System.* New York: Pergamon. Pp. 279–292.

Shamsie, Jalal. 1982. Anti-social adolescents: Our treatments are not working — Where do we go from here? *Annual Progress in Child Psychiatry & Child Development,* 7, 631–647.

Shrout, Patrick E., Michael Lyons, Bruce P. Dohrenwend, Andrew E. Skodol, Murray Solomon & Frederick Kass. 1988. Changing time frames on symptom inventories: Effects on the Psychiatric Epidemiology Research Interview. *Journal of Consulting & Clinical Psychology,* 56, 267–272.

Sila, Ante. 1972. Psychopathologic traits of perpetrators of felonious homicides. *Socijalna Psichijatrija,* 5, 3–81.

Silver, Jonathan M., Stuart C. Yudofsky & Robert E. Hales. 1987. Neuro- psychiatric aspects of traumatic brain injury. In Robert E. Hales & Stuart C. Yudofsky (eds.), *American Psychiatric Press Textbook of Neuropsychiatry.* Washington, DC: American Psychiatric Press. Pp. 179–190.

Simon, Robert I. 1987. *Clinical Psychiatry and the Law.* Washington, DC: American Psychiatric Press.

Sivak, Michael. 1983. Society's aggression level as a predictor of traffic fatality rate. *Journal of Safety Research,* 14, 93–99.

Smith, Lynda B., David E. Silber & Stephen A. Karp. 1988. Validity of the Megargee-Bohn MMPI typology with women incarcerated in a state prison. *Psychological Reports,* 62, 107–113.

Spellacy, Frank J. 1978. Neuropsychological discrimination between violent and nonviolent men. *Journal of Clinical Psychology,* 34, 49–52.

Spellacy, Frank J., & W.G. Brown. 1984. Prediction of recidivism in young offenders after brief institutionalization. *Journal of Clinical Psychology,* 40, 1070–1074.

Srole, Leo, Thomas S. Langer, Stanley T. Michael, Marvin K. Opler & Thomas A.C. Bennie. 1962. *Mental Health in the Metropolis.* New York: McGraw-Hill.

Srole, Leo, & Anita Kassen Fischer. 1986. The Midtown Manhattan longitudinal study: Aging, generations, and genders. In Myrna M. Weissman, Jerome K. Myers & Catherine E. Ross (eds.), *Community Surveys of Psychiatric Disorders.* New Brunswick, NJ: Rutgers University Press. Pp. 77–108.

Steadman, Henry J. 1982. A situational approach to violence. *International Journal of Law & Psychiatry,* 5, 171–186.

Steadman, Henry J., Marilyn J. Rogenstein, Robin L. MacAskill, & Ronald W. Manderscheid. 1988. A profile of mentally disordered offenders admitted to inpatient psychiatric services in the United States. *Law & Human Behavior,* 12, 91–99.

Stickney, Stonewall B. 1976. *Wyatt v. Stickney:* Background and post-mortem. In Stuart Golann and William J. Fremouw (eds.), *The Right to Treatment for Mental Patients.* New York: Irvington. Pp. 29–46.

Stone, Alan A. 1976. *Mental Health and Law: A System in Transition.* New York: Jason Aronson.

Stone, Alan A. 1984. *Law, Psychiatry, and Morality.* Washington, DC: American Psychiatric Press.

Stoudemire, G. Alan. 1987. Selected organic mental disorders. In Robert E. Hales & Stuart C. Yudofsky (eds.), *American Psychiatric Press Textbook of Neuropsychiatry.* Washington, DC: American Psychiatric Press. Pp. 125–140.

Swett, Chester, & Stuart C. Hartz. 1984. Antecedents of violent acts in a prison hospital. *American Journal of Social Psychiatry,* 4, 24–29.

Szymusik, A. 1972. Studies on the psychopathology of murderers. *Polish Medical Journal,* 11, 752–757.

Tardiff, Kenneth J. 1988. Violence. In John A. Talbott, Robert E. Hales & Stuart C. Yudofsky (eds.), *American Psychiatric Press Textbook of Psychiatry.* Washington, DC: American Psychiatric Press. Pp. 1037–1058.

Tarter, Ralph E., Andrea M. Hegedus & Arthur T. Alterman. 1983. Cognitive capacities of juvenile, violent, nonviolent, and sexual offenders. *Journal of Nervous & Mental Disease,* 171, 564–567.

Tarter, Ralph E., Andrea M. Hegedus, Nancy E. Winsten & Arthur I. Alterman. 1984. Neuropsychological, personality, and familial characteristics of physically abused delinquents. *Journal of the American Academy of Child Psychiatry,* 23, 668–674.

Taylor, Michael Alan, Frederick S. Sierles, & Richard Abrams. 1987. The neuropsychiatric evaluation. In Robert E. Hales & Stuart C. Yudofsky (eds.), *American Psychiatric Press Textbook of Neuropsychiatry.* Washington, DC: American Psychiatric Press. Pp. 3–16.

Taylor, Pamela J. 1986. Psychiatric disorder in London's life-sentenced offenders. *British Journal of Criminology,* 26, 63–78.

Teplin, Linda A. 1983. The criminalization of the mentally ill: Speculation in search of data. *Psychological Bulletin,* 94, 54–67.

Toborg, Mary A., & John P. Bellassai. 1987. *Assessment of Pretrial Urine Testing in the District of Columbia, I: Background and Description of the Urine Testing Program; IV: Analysis of Drug Use Among Arrestees.* Washington, DC: Toborg Associates.

Toch, Hans. 1975. *Men in Crisis: Human Breakdowns in Prison.* Chicago: Aldine.

Toch, Hans, Kenneth Adams & J. Douglas Grant. 1988. *Coping: Maladaptation in Prisons.* New Brunswick, NJ: Transaction.

Toch, Hans, Kenneth Adams & Ronald Greene. 1987. Ethnicity, disruptiveness, and emotional disorder among prison inmates. *Criminal Justice & Behavior,* 14, 93–109.

Torrey, E. Fuller. 1988. *Nowhere to Go: The Tragic Odyssey of the Homeless Mentally III.* New York: Harper & Row.

Torstensson, Marie. 1987. *Drug Abusers in a Metropolitan Cohort.* Stockholm: Department of Sociology, University of Stockholm.

Tuchfeld, Barry S., Richard R. Clayton & John A. Logan. 1982. Alcohol, drug use, and delinquent criminal behavior among male adolescents and young adults. *Journal of Drug Issues,* 12, 185–198.

Van Praag, H.M. 1988. Biological psychiatry audited. *Journal of Nervous & Mental Disease,* 176, 195–199.

Veneziano, Carol A. 1986. Prison inmates and consent to treatment: Problems and issues. *Law & Psychology Review,* 10, 129–146.

Veneziano, Carol A., & Louis Veneziano. 1986. Classification of adolescent offenders with the MMPI: An extension and cross-validation of the Megargee typology. *International Journal of Offender Therapy & Comparative Criminology,* 30, 11–23.

Vigderhous, Gideon. 1975. Suicide and homicide as causes of death and their relationship to life expectancy: A cross- national comparison. *Social Biology,* 22, 338–343.

Villanueva, Michael R., Deborah D. Roman & Michael R. Tuley. 1988. Determining forensic rehabilitation potential with the MMPI: Practical implications for residential treatment populations. *American Journal of Forensic Psychology,* 6, 27–35.

Virkkunen, Matti. 1974. Suicide linked to homicide. *Psychiatric Quarterly,* 48, 276–282.

Virkkunen, Matti. 1979. Alcoholism and antisocial personality. *Acta Psychiatrica Scandinavica,* 59, 493–501.

Virkkunen, Matti. 1982-*a*. Evidence for abnormal glucose tolerance test among violent offenders. *Neuropsychobiology,* 8, 30–34.

Virkkunen, Matti. 1982-*b*. Reactive hypoglycemic tendency among habitually violent offenders: A further study by means of the glucose tolerance test. *Neuropsychobiology,* 8, 35–40.

Virkkunen, Matti. 1983-*a*. Insulin secretion during the glucose tolerance test in antisocial personality. *British Journal of Psychiatry,* 142, 598–604.

Virkkunen, Matti. 1983-*b*. Serum cholesterol levels in homicidal offenders: A low cholesterol level is connected with a habitually violent tendency under the influence of alcohol. *Neuropsychobiology,* 10, 65–69.

Virkkunen, Matti. 1984. Reactive hypoglycemic tendency among arsonists. *Acta Psychiatrica Scandinavica,* 69, 445–452.

Virkkunen, Matti. 1985. Urinary free cortisol secretion in habitually violent offenders. *Acta Psychiatrica Scandinavica,* 72, 40–44.

Virkkunen, Matti. 1986. Insulin secretion during the glucose tolerance test among habitually violent and impulsive offenders. *Aggressive Behavior,* 12, 303–310.

Virkkunen, Matti, & M.O. Huttunen. 1982. Evidence for abnormal glucose tolerance test among violent offenders. *Neuropsychobiology,* 8, 30–34.

Virkkunen, Matti, & Eila Kallilo. 1987. Low blood glucose nadir in the glucose tolerance test and homicidal spouse abuse. *Aggressive Behavior,* 13, 59–66.

Virkkunen, Matti, & S. Narvanen. 1987. Plasma insulin, tryptophan, and serotonin levels during the glucose tolerance test among habitually violent and impulsive offenders. *Neuropsychobiology,* 17, 19–23.

Virkkunen, Matti, Arto Nuutila & Simo Huusko. 1976. Effect of brain injury on social adaptability: Longitudinal study on frequency of criminality. *Acta Psychiatrica Scandinavica*, 53, 168–172.

Virkkunen, Matti, David F. Horrobin, Douglas K. Jenkins & Mehar S. Manku. 1987. Plasma phospholipid essentially fatty acids and prostaglandins in alcoholic, habitually violent, and impulsive offenders. *Biological Psychiatry*, 22, 1087–1096.

Virkkunen, Matti, Arto Nuutila, Frederick K. Goodwin, & Markku Linnoila. 1987. Cerebrospinal fluid monamine metabolite levels in male arsonists. *Archives of General Psychiatry*, 44, 241–247.

Virkkunen, Matti, Judith de Jong, John J. Bartko & Frederick K. Goodwin. 1989. Relationship of psychobiological variables to recidivism in violent offenders and impulsive fire setters: A follow-up study. *Archives of General Psychiatry*, 46, 600–603.

von Hirsch, Andrew. 1976. *Doing Justice: The Choice of Punishments*. New York: Hill & Wang.

von Hirsch, Andrew. 1985. *Past or Future Crimes: Deservedness and Dangerousness in the Sentencing of Criminals*. New Brunswick, NJ: Rutgers University Press.

von Hirsch, Andrew. 1988. *Federal Sentencing Guidelines: The United States and Canadian Schemes Compared*. New York: Center for Research in Crime & Justice, School of Law, New York University.

Walkey, Frank J., & D. Ross Gilmour. 1984. The relationship between interpersonal distance and violence in imprisoned offenders. *Criminal Justice & Behavior*, 11, 331–340.

Walters, Glenn D. 1986-*a*. Correlates of the Megargee criminal classification system: A military correctional setting. *Criminal Justice & Behavior*, 13, 19–32.

Walters, Glenn D. 1986-*b*. Screening for psychopathology in groups and black and white prison inmates by means of the MMPI. *Journal of Personality Assessment*, 50, 257–264.

Walters, Glenn D., Thomas A. Scrapansky & Glenn A. Marlow. 1986. The emotionally disturbed military criminal offender: Identification, background, and institutional adjustment. *Criminal Justice & Behavior*, 13, 261–285.

Walters, Glenn D., Thomas W. White & Roger L. Greene. 1988. Use of the MMPI to identify malingering and exaggeration of psychiatric symptomatology in male prison inmates. *Journal of Consulting & Clinical Psychology*, 56, 111–117.

Warheit, George J., Roger A. Bell, John J. Schwab, and Joanne M. Buhl. 1986. An epidemiologic assessment of mental health problems in the southeastern United States. In Myrna M. Weissman, Jerome K. Myers & Catherine E. Ross (eds.), *Community Surveys of Psychiatric Disorders*. New Brunswick, NJ: Rutgers University Press. Pp. 191–208.

Washington, Pat, & Ronald J. Diamond. 1985. Prevalence of mental illness among women incarcerated in five California county jails. *Research in Community Mental Health*, 5, 33–41.

Weissman, Myrna M., Jerome K. Myers & Pamela S. Harding. 1978. Psychiatric disorders in a U.S. urban community. *American Journal of Psychiatry*, 135, 459–462.

Weissman, Myrna M., Jerome K. Myers & Catherine E. Ross. 1986. Community studies in psychiatric epidemiology. In Myrna M. Weissman, Jerome K. Myers & Catherine E. Ross (eds.), *Community Surveys of Psychiatric Disorders*. New Brunswick, NJ: Rutgers University Press. Pp. 1 -19.

Welte, John W., & Brenda A. Miller. 1987. Alcohol use by violent and property offenders. *Drug & Alcohol Dependence*, 19, 313–324.

West, Donald J., & Alexander Walk, eds. 1977. *Daniel McNaughton: His Trial and the Aftermath*. Ashford, Kent: Royal College of Psychiatrists.

Wettstein, Robert M. 1987. Legal aspects of neuropsychiatry. In Robert E. Hales and Stuart C. Yudofsky (eds.), *American Psychiatric Press Textbook of Neuropsychiatry*. Washington, DC: American Psychiatric Press. Pp. 451–463.

Wettstein, Robert M. 1988. Psychiatry and the law. In John A. Talbott, Robert E. Hales & Stuart C. Yudofsky (eds.), *American Psychiatric Press Textbook of Psychiatry*. Washington, DC: American Psychiatric Press. Pp. 1059–1084.

Whatmore, George B., & Daniel R. Kohli. 1974. *The Physiopathology and Treatment of Functional Disorder*. New York: Grune & Stratton.

Wheaton, Blair. 1982. Uses and abuses of the Langner Index: A Re-examination of findings on psychological and psychophysiological distress. In David Mechanic (ed.), *Symptoms, Illness Behavior, and Help-Seeking*. New York: Prodist/Neale Watson. Pp. 25–53.

Whitman, Steven, Tina E. Coleman, Cecil Patmon,Bindu T. Desai, Robert Cohen & Lambert N. King. 1984. Epilepsy in prison: Elevated prevalence and no relationship to violence. *Neurology*, 34, 775–782.

Wilbanks, William. 1982. Fatal accidents, suicide, and homicide: Are they related? *Victimology*, 7, 213–217.

Wilcox, David E. 1985. The relationship of mental illness to homicide. *American Journal of Forensic Psychiatry*, 6, 3–15.

Williams, Janet B.W., Jean Endicott & Robert L. Spitzer. 1986. Some biometric contributions to assessment: PSS, CAPPS, SADS-L/RDC, and DSM-III. In Myrna M. Weissman, Jerome K. Myers & Catherine E. Ross (eds.), *Community Surveys of Psychiatric Disorders*. New Brunswick, NJ: Rutgers University Press. Pp. 377–402.

Wilmotte, J.N., & J.P. Plat-Mendlewicz. 1973. Epidemiology of suicidal behavior in one thousand Belgian prisoners. In Bruce L. Danto (ed.), *Jail House Blues: Studies of Suicidal Behavior in Jail and Prison*. Detroit: Epic. Pp. 57–82.

Wilson, James Q., & Richard J. Herrnstein. 1985. *Crime & Human Nature: The Definitive Study of the Causes of Crime*. New York: Simon & Schuster.

Wilson, Margo, & Martin Daly. 1985. Competitiveness, risk taking, and violence: The young male syndrome. *Ethology & Sociobiology*, 6, 59–73.

Windle, Charles, Paul J. Poppen, James W. Thompson & Kevin Marvelle. 1988 Types of patients served by various providers of outpatient care in CMHCs. *Journal of Consulting & Clinical Psychology*, 56, 457–463.

Wish, Eric D. 1990. Drug testing. In Larry J. Siegel (ed.), *American Justice.* St. Paul, MN: West. Pp. 109–113.

Wish, Eric D., & Joyce Ann O'Neil. 1989. Drug use forecasting (DUF) research update. *Research in Action: Drug Use Forecasting.* National Institute of Justice, U.S. Department of Justice, September 1989.

Wish, Eric D., Elizabeth Brady & Mary Cuadrado. 1986. *Urine Testing of Arrestees: Findings from Manhattan.* New York: Narcotic and Drug Research, Inc.

Wolfe, David A., John A. Fairbank, Jeffrey A. Kelly & Andrew S. Bradlyn. 1983. Child abusive parents' physiological responses to stressful and non-stressful behavior in children. *Behavioral Assessment*, 5, 363–371.

Wolfgang, Marvin E. 1958. *Patterns in Criminal Homicide.* Philadelphia: University of Pennsylvania Press.

Wolfgang, Marvin E., & Franco Ferracuti. 1967. *The Subculture of Violence.* London: Tavistock.

Wood, Rodger Llewellyn. 1987. *Brain Injury Rehabilitation: A Neurobehavioral Approach.* Rockville, MD: Aspen.

Wormith, J. Stephen. 1984. The controversy over the effects of long-term incarceration. *Canadian Journal of Criminology*, 26, 423–437.

Wormith, J. Stephen, & C.S. Goldstone. 1984. Clinical and statistical prediction of recidivism. *Criminal Justice & Behavior*, 11, 3–34.

Wright, Kevin N. 1991. The violent and the victimized in the male prison. *Journal of Offender Rehabilitation*, 16, 201–220.

Yeudall, Lorne T., & D. Fromm-Auch. 1979. Neuropsychological impairments in various psychopathological populations. In John Gruzelier & Pierre Flor-Henry (eds.), *Hemisphere Asymmetries of Function in Psychopathology.* Amsterdam: Elsevier/North Holland Biomedical Press. Pp. 401 428.

Yeudall, Lorne T., Orestes Fedora & DaLee Fromm. 1987. A neuropsychological theory of persistent criminality: Implications for assessment and treatment. *Advances in Forensic Psychology & Psychiatry*, 2, 119–191.

Yohman, J. Robert, Kim W. Schaeffer & Oscar A. Parsons. 1988. Cognitive retraining in alcoholic men. *Journal of Consulting & Clinical Psychology*, 56, 67–72.

Zager, Lynne D. 1988. The MMPI-based criminal classification system: A review, current status, and future directions. *Criminal Justice & Behavior*, 15, 39–57.

Index